Prostate Cancer and the Man You Love

Prostate Cancer and the Man You Love

Supporting and Caring for Your Partner

Anne Katz

ROWMAN & LITTLEFIELD PUBLISHERS, INC.

Lanham • Boulder • New York • Toronto • Plymouth, UK

Published by Rowman & Littlefield Publishers, Inc.
A wholly owned subsidiary of The Rowman & Littlefield Publishing Group, Inc.
4501 Forbes Boulevard, Suite 200, Lanham, Maryland 20706
www.rowman.com

10 Thornbury Road, Plymouth PL6 7PP, United Kingdom

British Library Cataloguing in Publication Information Available

Library of Congress Cataloging-in-Publication Data
Katz, Anne (Anne Jennifer), 1958–
Prostate cancer and the man you love : supporting and caring for your partner / Anne Katz.
    p. cm.
 ISBN 978-1-4422-1452-1 (cloth : alk. paper) — ISBN 978-1-4422-1454-5 (ebook)
 1. Cancer—Patients—Family relationships. 2. Men—Sexual behavior. 3. Cancer—Patients—Rehabilitation. 4. Sex (Psychology) I. Title.
 RC262.K3594 2012
 616.99'463—dc23   2012010578

∞™ The paper used in this publication meets the minimum requirements of American National Standard for Information Sciences—Permanence of Paper for Printed Library Materials, ANSI/NISO Z39.48-1992.

Printed in the United States of America

Acknowledgment

For and about everything
Alan

Contents

Preface

$\mathcal{F}$or the past eight years I have spent part of all my working days talking to couples about prostate cancer. Part of my role in my position as clinical nurse specialist at CancerCare Manitoba is to help the man and his partner make a decision about treatment that is right for him (and the couple) in the context of their life together and that is based on their values and beliefs. It has long been recognized that when men are involved in the process of treatment decision making after a diagnosis of prostate cancer, they are more satisfied with the treatment and experience less regret. I always insist that men bring their partner with them, and they mostly do. There are always some men who think that this is their problem to solve on their own, but I tell them that the disease and its treatment will affect them as a couple and that the presence of their partner is required.

And so they arrive at the appointed time, and mostly I see a couple whose life has been turned upside down by the diagnosis. I can usually tell them three things that I am certain of: that things will get better, that they have a lot to learn and that the learning journey will be an interesting one, and that they will get through this crisis and they will come out stronger as a couple, even when the long-term outlook is not good.

This book contains the long version of what they have to learn. Each chapter describes a unique aspect of prostate cancer, from the nuts and bolts of diagnosis to the sensitive topic of end-of-life care. It is written for and about the partner/spouse of the man with prostate cancer because no book exists that addresses this topic from that perspective. There are many books for the man with prostate cancer, but the partner is an aside, a supportive player to the man. I wanted to put the partner front and center while not forgetting that it is the man with the disease. Each chapter is punctuated by stories of couples who are on this journey. These are not real couples but rather composite characters who experience many of the real challenges that I have witnessed in my practice. There are old and young couples, gay and straight couples, and couples from different ethnic and cultural backgrounds. I hope that you empathize with them and perhaps even see yourselves in their stories.

I have purposely used the term *spouse/partner* instead of *husband* for a couple of reasons. First, there are many gay men with this disease, and they remain largely invisible in a medical world that ignores them and a society that does not recognize same-sex marriage (although that is changing). And there are many couples who are not married in the civil or religious sense, and so my choice of words is deliberate. My intent was to be inclusive and not to offend.

• 1 •

Introduction

$\mathcal{Y}$ou likely bought this book or were given it because your partner or spouse has been diagnosed with prostate cancer. No doubt your world has been turned upside down by this news. It's now time for you both to start learning about this disease so that you can be prepared for what might come next. So sit back, take a deep breath, and start reading. We're going to start with the basics of prostate cancer in this chapter and move from there to the details, chapter by chapter.

WHERE AND WHAT IS THE PROSTATE GLAND?

The prostate gland is a walnut-shaped organ that lies just beneath the bladder, deep in the pelvis. A tube called the urethra runs through it, taking urine and semen to the outside of the body through the penis. The prostate lies in front of the rectum and can be felt through the wall of the rectum—the digital rectal examination is done to feel the posterior surface of the prostate gland and is the only way that it can be felt by physical examination.

Two wing-shaped pieces are attached to the prostate gland and lie slightly above and behind the gland; these are the seminal vesicles that contain some fluid that is added to the fluid that the prostate itself makes. This fluid (called seminal fluid) joins the sperm that are produced by the testicles to make up the semen. The seminal fluids nourish and protect the sperm and provide the fluid medium for semen to be expelled and begin their search for an egg inside a woman's body. The main purpose of the prostate gland is to produce the seminal fluids and to contract and expel semen during ejaculation.

1

The prostate gland has an outside capsule; this is important to know about because you may hear the doctor say that the cancer has not spread outside the capsule (this is good) or that there is extracapsular extension (the cancer has moved outside the capsule; this is not so good). Running on either side of the prostate gland are two neurovascular bundles—these contain blood vessels and the nerves responsible for erections; you'll hear much more about these later.

WHAT IS THE PSA?

Prostate tissue produces a protein called prostate-specific antigen (PSA), and measuring the level of PSA in the blood has become the mainstay of early detection of prostate cancer and is the source of a lot of controversy. Most of us believe, because we are told this daily by the media as well as friends and relatives and our health-care providers, that the sooner you find out you have cancer the better, and the sooner you start treatment the more likely the cancer will be cured or at least kept in check. This is why there is so much importance placed on screening for cancer; think about Pap tests for cervical cancer in women as well as mammography for breast cancer. Both of these are screening tests. The screening test for prostate cancer is the PSA test, and there is much controversy about its usefulness and accuracy.

Prior to the introduction of the PSA test in the mid-1990s, most men who were diagnosed with prostate cancer were identified in one of two ways. The first was men who presented to their doctors with evidence of widespread cancer. On examination, these men would have a large, hard prostate, further evidence of advanced prostate cancer, and probably were also having significant urinary problems. They usually had a history of frequent urination, and this may have progressed to urinary obstruction, where the tube that carries urine out of the body (the urethra) had been compressed by the enlarged prostate gland. These men would already have experienced a spreading of the cancer to the bones and so might have what we call a pathological fracture, a break of a bone that occurs without any significant trauma, such as a fractured rib on coughing. There was often not much that could be done for these men other than treating their pain from the cancer in the bones and perhaps inserting a catheter into the bladder to allow for the urine to be drained.

The second way that prostate cancer was diagnosed was in men who were experiencing urinary difficulties as a result of an enlarged prostate. These men would have a surgical procedure called a transurethral resection of the prostate (TURP), often referred to as a "Roto-Rooter" operation, where tissue would be scraped out along the urethra where it passes through the prostate gland. This tissue would then be examined by a pathologist and the presence of cancer reported. Depending on their age and other factors, treatment would be offered to these men, many of whom would later die of something other than prostate cancer.

Then in the 1970s, a protein called PSA (prostate specific antigen) was discovered by a professor of immunology, Dr. Richard Ablin. A test to detect this protein was developed and introduced in the 1990s. Since then, the use of this screening test has been accepted widely, despite a lack of evidence of the test's ability to identify those with prostate cancer. A raised PSA level leads to more invasive testing, such as a biopsy where tissue is taken from the prostate itself and examined, and to a lot of anxiety. Because of the widespread use of PSA screening, hundreds of thousands of men are diagnosed with prostate cancer, and many of them do not need treatment and will die of something else; but once they know they have cancer, they and their loved ones want treatment immediately and aggressively, and treatment may in fact not be necessary at all. You will read more about this in chapter 4.

The diagnosis of prostate cancer can only be made after a prostate biopsy in which tissue is taken from the gland itself. The PSA test is a screening test and reflects the amount of a protein that is produced by the prostate. The PSA level may be increased because of infection in the prostate, use of over-the-counter drugs such as ibuprofen, and enlargement of the prostate as a man ages. Ironically, the true usefulness of the PSA test lies in its ability to identify the presence of recurrent prostate cancer after treatment.

WHAT ABOUT THE PROSTATE BIOPSY?

The PSA cannot tell if a man has cancer or not. The only way to do that is to take samples of the prostate itself and look at them under a microscope. Cancer cells look a certain way and are different from normal, healthy cells; this is true for all kinds of cancer. A prostate biopsy is performed to obtain tissue from the prostate to see if there is cancer present. It is an office procedure that is done while the patient is awake, but it is suggested that the man have someone with him to drive him home just in case he doesn't feel well.

An ultrasound probe is inserted into the rectum, and a local anesthetic is injected close to the nerves around the prostate. Then samples, usually twelve to fourteen, are taken from the prostate and sent for evaluation by a pathologist. The procedure should not be painful, although many men find the probe itself uncomfortable. The pathologist looks at the samples under a microscope, and when cancer is seen, a numerical value, called the Gleason score, is assigned to each sample. The Gleason score is a measure of the aggressiveness of the cancer and is used as part of the process to decide what treatment is appropriate for the individual man.

The Gleason score ranges from 6/10 to 10/10, with the higher number representing aggressive cancer. The number is assigned based on how much the cancer cells look like normal prostate cells; this is described as the "differentiation" of the cells. The Gleason score is based on two numbers that are added together. The first number represents the appearance of the cancer cells that occupy the greatest volume in that sample, and the second number reflects the appearance of the second greatest volume of cancer cells in that same sample. The Gleason scores can be described as low risk (Gleason 6), intermediate risk (Gleason 7), and high risk (Gleason 8, 9, and 10). You may read in some books or pamphlets about Gleason scores less than 6; anything under 6 is regarded as normal and so is not reported as being cancer.

Some men experience bleeding from the rectum after the procedure, but this should stop within a few hours. If it persists, the man should contact his urologist. Men are usually instructed to take antibiotics for a day or two before and after the biopsy to prevent infection. The urine may be bloodstained for a few days to a few weeks. His ejaculate (or semen) may be discolored for a month or more after the procedure.

The results of the biopsy should be communicated to the man as soon as they are received, as he (and his partner/spouse) may be quite anxious. Some physicians do this over the phone if no cancer is found but will want to see the man in person if cancer is present. Others will tell the patient on the phone that he has prostate cancer and ask to see the man for a discussion about treatment (see chapter 3) at a later date. It is important that you (or a close friend or family member) go with him to all his appointments, but especially the one where the results of a biopsy are discussed. We know that after someone hears the words "You have cancer," they are able to focus on only about 10 percent of the information that comes next. And there is often a lot of information that is provided after the diagnosis. Some people say that after they heard these words, it was like a train went through their head, and all they could hear was noise that shut out the words of the physician.

WHAT IS THE CLINICAL STAGE?

The clinical stage is determined by what the doctor feels when he/she does a digital rectal examination. This is not a very accurate test as it depends on the experience of the doctor and is of course subjective. Stage T1 describes a normal feeling prostate with cancer identified on biopsy. Stage T2 refers to cancer that is confined to the prostate gland and is further described as T2a (cancer in 50 percent or less of one lobe of the gland), T2b (cancer in more than 50 percent of one lobe), or T2c (cancer in both lobes). In stage T3, the cancer extends outside the capsule, and stage T4 means that the cancer is outside the prostate and is stuck to other organs.

After surgery, the pathologist may also describe the cancer in relation to lymph node involvement (N0 means that no cancer was found in the lymph nodes, and N1 or more means that one or more lymph nodes had cancer). The letter M in a pathology report refers to the presence or absence of metastases (distant spread).

WHAT ABOUT OTHER TESTS?

There are other tests, usually imaging tests that can be used to help in the decision making for the treatment of prostate cancer. The most commonly used imaging tests in prostate cancer are CT scans, bone scans, and MRI scans. Bone scans should only be used in men who have high-risk prostate cancer (Gleason scores of 8, 9, or 10) and/or PSA levels above 20 ng/nl. The purpose of having a bone scan is to look for evidence that the cancer has (or has not) spread to the bones. You will read more about metastatic prostate cancer later in this book (chapters 8 and 9), and if the cancer has spread to the bone, different treatments will be prescribed for the man.

CT scans are used to look for enlarged lymph nodes in the pelvis. There is not much value from this in men with low-risk prostate cancer, so the benefits are debatable. CT scans do not tell us much about the prostate cancer itself and so should be used sparingly in men with low-risk prostate cancer. They may be of more value in men with advanced prostate cancer and are used as part of the planning process for external beam radiation.

MRI scans of the prostate are done with a special coil that is inserted in the rectum. It can be useful in telling us if the cancer has spread outside the prostate capsule or into the seminal vesicles. Clear guidelines for when MRI scans should be done have not been developed, but they are still done, often to put the patient's mind at rest even when they do not add information that would influence treatment decision making. A newer kind of MRI, spectroscopic magnetic resonance (MR-S) is not yet widely available but may add information about the metabolic characteristics of the cancer and will likely be useful for guiding radiation therapy to specific areas of the prostate.

ProstaScint scans use special radioactive molecules for identifying prostate cancer cells inside and outside the prostate gland. The use of this scan has been controversial, with early use not showing any benefit over traditional tests and scans. The use of ProstaScint scans is not routine, and you should be wary of anyone who suggests that this test must be done.

It is increasingly recognized that we have to be more careful in our use of these tests because they all expose people to doses of radiation that themselves can be dangerous to one's health. Over the course of a lifetime, repeated exposure to radiation from these imaging tests can increase the risk of developing cancer, so they must be used carefully and only when they add information about the disease, not "just to be sure" or "just to check." Having a questioning attitude is a good one for all imaging studies because of the risk from additional radiation exposure. When a doctor suggests additional scanning, asking why the test needs to be done and what information the test will add to the clinical management of the disease is a good strategy. At best, there may be no good reason for the test to be done; at worst, the test may be of no use but may cause potential long-term harm. Remember that the doctor may own the testing facility and may be making a lot of money from sending patients for tests that they don't need.

REACTIONS AND COPING

Prostate cancer has often been called a couple's disease, in part because the spouse or partner's reaction and adjustment to the diagnosis is critical to how the man himself will react and adjust to the diagnosis. Distress in response to the diagnosis or progression of the cancer is shared; however, studies have shown that in prostate cancer the distress of the partner/spouse is often greater than that of the man.[1] Partners often try and protect the man by not sharing their feelings and worries with him. This is quite common and is intended to help, but it mostly increases your distress and is regarded as maladaptive by the experts.[2] Prostate cancer doesn't pick its targets—it can happen to couples who have a great relationship and to those who don't; in strained relationships, the partner may actively avoid the man, minimize his illness and its consequences, and be falsely cheerful. This usually ends with the man feeling rejected and abandoned.

Having a positive and supportive coping style results in feelings of mutual trust, reliability, and a perception that you will both get through whatever you have to face. This also helps to decrease distress and sustains the relationship through challenging times. Couples often experience something called posttraumatic growth, where priorities are changed as a result of the cancer experience and benefits are seen. These positive changes are a result of information seeking, learning to see the positive in situations, and mutual emotional support.[3]

Depending on your age when he is diagnosed, response to the cancer and the effects that it can have on your life will differ. In couples in middle age (fifties and sixties), prostate cancer interrupts what should be a happy and worry-free time of life. At this age, many couples have launched their own children and have fewer financial stressors. Many couples at this stage are planning their retirement and looking forward to some leisure. Cancer at this stage of life may prompt early retirements and cause financial stress. The treatments for the cancer affect daily life and normal day-to-day functioning. The side effects on sexual intimacy for the couple are often seen as something that the couple expected later in life and not in this, the prime of their lives.

For couples in their late sixties and early seventies, this is a time when retirement has usually happened and the couple is making the transition to another way of life. The physical changes associated with aging often start in this phase of life, so illness is not entirely unexpected; however it can and does interfere with what the couple may have planned for their retirement years. This is often a stage in which couples evaluate their life plans and achievements and often feel that they have done what they wanted to do, so while illness is never welcomed, it is balanced with a life well lived and enjoyed for many.

For older couples (mid-seventies and older), prostate cancer occurs at a time when illness may be expected; however this does not lessen its impact. The older the man, the more likely it is that his recovery will be slow, and coping with a complex medical problem may seem overwhelming. The partner/spouse may be dealing with his or her own physical health issues, which can make support challenging. On the other hand, friends and family of a similar age may also be dealing with illness, so there is support and experience from others, and ill health may not come as such a shock.

CHANGES IN THE RELATIONSHIP

Most of what we know about prostate cancer in couples is based on our experience and research with heterosexual couples. There is a limited amount of information about what happens to gay men when one is diagnosed with prostate cancer. Two useful books about this are referenced in the bibliography section of this book.[4]

Most of the research done about relationship changes has been in older couples where traditional roles are the norm. This may change over time as societal norms change (e.g., both partners working outside the home). In an illuminating study of four hundred couples over eight years, 113 female partners spoke poignantly about the changes in their relationships after prostate cancer.[5] They describe coping with their husband's cancer while the rest of their life was taking place. They had to learn new things (managing finances and dealing with household repairs) while trying to balance their regular activities with illness-related events. These everyday activities (seeing friends, getting exercise, going to the hairdresser) were seen as important for their emotional health. They found that their husband's illness interfered with their usual socializing and outside relationships. Many of the women reported that their faith and prayer were very important to them and helped them cope.

The women were challenged by the cancer itself, and many reported feeling that they were waiting for the next (bad) thing to happen. They worried a lot about what their mate was going through—his pain, how to help, anxiety about what the results of future blood tests would mean—at the same time as they worried about what would happen to them if and when he died. They talked about "silent suffering," and part of this was the loss of an active and pleasurable sex life as a result of treatment. They remarked on the happy memories they had of their previous life while at the same time struggling to find alternative ways of being close to their husbands now that sex was no longer a part of their lives. Some of the women interviewed blamed age for the lack of sexual interest and activity in their relationship, while others struggled to accept that the effects of the treatment were causing the man's lack of interest in them as a sexual partner. Some of the women described growing apart from their husbands, and this was not helped by challenges in their communication.

Many of the women said that their husbands didn't want to talk about what was happening, and so to avoid making things worse the women didn't try to bring up the subject. For some women, this lack of willingness to talk things through felt like a betrayal. This need to pussyfoot around their husband's feelings was a significant stressor for the women. But other women used humor and patience to deal with the changes they saw in their partners and tried to cope by exercising, eating well, and trying different kinds of alternative therapies.

SO WHAT CAN *YOU* DO?

Every couple is different—and there is no one-size-fits-all approach to how you and your partner/spouse are going to respond to the diagnosis and cope with what comes after. We generally react to challenges in life as we always have—so if he has withdrawn and not wanted to talk about things in the past, then that is likely how he will react to the diagnosis. And the same can be said for you—if you generally reach out and seek support, then you will do so again now. The problem is that the person you may always have asked for support (your partner/spouse) is the patient in this case and may not be able to support you.

You have an important role to play in this journey. We know that partners/spouses often become the primary health advocates for their partners and that they are also the primary sources of support for men experiencing a health crisis or ongoing health issues. You are also the one person who is most likely to help him make a treatment decision and then cope with the side effects if and when they arise. It is also common for partners/spouses to seek out all the health information they can about the disease, share that information with the man, and then allow him to make his decision.[6]

WHAT COMES NEXT . . .

Reading this book is the first step in your search for knowledge about prostate cancer. It will provide you with evidence-based information about prostate cancer, the various treatments for this disease, and strategies for coping with it. There are also good quality websites with accurate information that you can peruse for additional information; the chapters in this book contain some suggestions for websites dedicated to supporting you and your partner/spouse. So turn the page and let's start . . .

What Do We Do?

Confronting the Challenges of Diagnosis

*T*he period of time when a man waits for the results of his biopsy can be very tense and full of anxiety. And once the diagnosis is made, there is a lot of new medical information that has to be learned and understood to help the man make an appropriate treatment decision.

PLAYING THE WAITING GAME

For some men, worrying about prostate cancer begins long before being tested for the presence of cancer. Men with a family history of prostate cancer may be anxious for many years that they too will be diagnosed in the future. Each and every time they have a PSA test, they may be scared that it will show that they have cancer. Remember that the PSA test is a *screening* test and is not a test to detect cancer; only a biopsy will do that. They may also worry that what happened to men in their family will happen to them. So if their father died of prostate cancer, they may assume that the same fate awaits them. There is no evidence that what happened to a relative will happen to any man. And if the relative was treated many years ago, his path may be irrelevant, as treatments have changed over time and are much better now than they were years ago, and most men diagnosed with prostate cancer today are identified as a result of an abnormal PSA test and so are diagnosed very early in the disease process.

Even with this worry, many men have very little knowledge about prostate cancer. In one study,[1] 80 percent of respondents did not know the function of the prostate, and almost half did not know that prostate cancer is the most common internal cancer in men (second only to skin cancer). More than a third did not know about the treatments for this cancer, and more than half did not know about the side effects of the treatments for this disease. Another study[2] suggests that men may have poor recall of events around the time of diagnosis. In this study, over four hundred men with prostate cancer were asked about the testing they had leading up to the diagnosis of cancer. Less than 20 percent recalled having a biopsy! Recall was worse the older the man, with those of seventy years of age remembering the least about having a PSA test, a digital rectal exam, or ultrasound and biopsy.

Waiting for biopsy results can be a very stressful time, and it's normal to play a "what-if" game in your head and heart. What if it's cancer? What are we going to do? What can I do to help him? Why won't he talk about what he is thinking and feeling? This is one of the reasons this book was written—to help you support the man you love and care for.

For men whose biopsy is negative, meaning that they don't have prostate cancer, the worry may continue after the results of the biopsy are known. In one study, 26 percent of men with a raised PSA level but normal biopsy result continued to worry about prostate cancer one year after the biopsy, and almost half of them stated that their wife or partner was concerned as well.[3] As you will see in the following chapters of this book, often the partner of the man is even more distressed than the man himself.

Other men don't tell their partners that they are even having a biopsy! While this may be hard to imagine, some men think that this is their problem to deal with and that if the news is not good, they'll tell their spouse or partner at the time. This is likely to lead to a very sad and confused spouse with perhaps some anger too.

John is fifty-four years old and finally went to see his family doctor after his wife Margie had nagged him for about nine months. He found out that his blood pressure was high, and he had to have a couple of samples of blood drawn. He was a little surprised to receive a call from his doctor to tell him that his PSA was raised and that he was being referred to see a urologist. He went to that appointment two weeks later and was even more shocked when the nurse told him he was having a biopsy of his prostate. He signed some forms, and the next thing he knew, he was lying on a table with something hard in his rectum. After ten minutes of intense embarrassment and twelve snaps of what the doctor called "the gun," he went home. He didn't want to worry Margie, so he said nothing and avoided having sex because the nurse had told him that his semen was going to be discolored. A week later, a week during which he hardly slept a wink, the urologist's office called and told him to come in for the last appointment of the day the following Friday. What did this mean?

He went to the appointment that Friday at 4:30 and came home a different man. He wasn't sure just what he'd been told, but the words "You have cancer" were there, and they rang in his head like an alarm. The rest was just noise; he saw the doctor's mouth moving and he was aware of his heart thumping in his chest, but that was all. What was he going to tell Margie? How was he going to tell her? He didn't know where to begin.

"I HAVE CANCER"

These are likely the worst words any spouse or partner wants to hear. If you didn't go with your spouse or partner to the appointment when he was told the results of the biopsy, or if you didn't listen in on the phone call with the urologist, you probably knew from the moment you saw his face that the news wasn't good. So what do you do?

There's no right or wrong way to react to this information. Your reaction will reflect your shock and pain, and that's okay. Only you know how best to cope with this, and how both of you have reacted to adversity in the past will inform what happens this time. For some couples, one individual has to be strong so that the other can be weak. That may be right for you, and you may have to hide your feelings from him in order to support him and get him through this difficult initial stage. For other couples, you may be the one to show your emotions while he is stoic. This is not the time to try to be someone other than who you are—pretending to be strong and not letting him know how you feel may not be the best thing. On the other hand, perhaps he needs you to express your sadness and shock so that he can support you and deal with his own feelings at another time. Every couple, and individual, is different.

You may be more distressed about this than the man is himself. This may sound strange, but think about a time when you had to face an illness or other challenge. It is sometimes easier to just put your head down and do what needs to be done; your spouse or partner has to watch you go through it, and that can be more difficult. Having a baby is like that—a woman in labor has a job to do; she has to have that baby one way or the other. The partner or spouse may find it very difficult to watch the woman in the throes of a contraction or pushing the baby out. The woman has to do the hard work, whereas the partner has to watch and empathize if he/she can. So don't be surprised if you seem more anxious or upset than your spouse or partner. It's not that he isn't worried; he just has a job to do now that he knows.

There are certain factors that may exacerbate the distress that a partner feels when a man is diagnosed with prostate cancer. These include lack of information, fear of the unknown, fear of what the future holds, and concerns about treatment. This is yet another reason why it is so important for you to go with the man to all of his appointments. It is there that you will learn more about the cancer and what lies ahead in terms of treatment and prognosis. Knowing this can help to prevent or at least alleviate some of your distress.[4]

There is evidence from research[5] that men who confront their illness in a direct way, emotionally or instrumentally, adapt better both psychologically and physically. So the man who doesn't try to avoid the topic or what comes next and who is active in making decisions about treatment will fare better psychologically in the long run than the man who tries to avoid dealing with his emotions and delays treatment decisions. Coping can also affect physical factors; men who try to put a positive spin on what they are experiencing (for example, prostate cancer when treated has a high survival rate) and who try to solve problems in an effective manner (for example, not waiting for the doctor's office to call to give them an appointment but rather calling themselves and getting the soonest appointment) tend to experience less fatigue than men who are more negative in outlook and more passive in problem solving.

How the man copes with the initial stress of diagnosis sets the stage for how he copes with the rest of his journey with prostate cancer. Men who don't cope well in the beginning tend to face more challenges during and after treatment, and this can have a negative impact on disease progression. Men who use avoidant coping mechanisms such as denial and disengagement ("I'm not going to deal with this; it'll all work out in the end") adapt poorly. Men who adapt emotionally in a positive way tend to do better in the long run; they tend to be optimistic ("It's going to be just fine, dear") and also seek out support that helps them cope ("I met this man who had surgery too, and he's just as good as he was before"). There do seem to be some differences related to age, however, with younger men experiencing more distress than their older counterparts, but they do seek out support more and tend to be more optimistic than older men with prostate cancer.

Christine could remember exactly what she was doing when her husband Bill called her that December afternoon. She was baking brownies in their winter-sun-filled kitchen; she had put them in the oven just twenty minutes before, and she was wiping down the countertops. The phone rang, and she held it between her head and shoulder as she continued to clean. The next thing she knew, the phone clattered to the floor and she could hear Bill's voice coming from where it landed on the floor: "Honey, are you there? Chris, what happened? Are you there? Chris?"

He came home soon after that. The timer on the oven was still buzzing, but the brownies sat on the kitchen counter. Chris was in the study, sitting in the office chair, staring into space.

"Honey, Chris, it's going to be okay. I promise. Chris? Are you okay?"

Bill's face was white, and Chris could see that his jaw was clenched. She wasn't sure what to say or do. Nothing had prepared her for this.

"I don't know if I'm okay. I don't know anything anymore. . . . How did this happen? Why? Why you?" Her voice sounded strange to him, as if she was talking through a straw.

Bill took a deep breath. "Remember, I told you I had to have some tests? I played it down because I was kind of scared. Anyway, that's in the past. The reality is I have prostate cancer. The doctor said it's early, it hasn't spread, and the outlook is good. But I have to have surgery."

Surgery! Her Bill had always been the healthy one. He'd watched her deal with the arthritis that ran in her family, and he'd been strong and supportive for her. How was she going to help him? How could she help him? She felt lost, and this time she wasn't sure that Bill could help her.

COPING WITH THE DIAGNOSIS

There is no doubt that a diagnosis of prostate cancer causes significant distress. Because most men are diagnosed today as a result of PSA screening, they tend to have very early-stage disease (which is a good thing) but they don't have any symptoms of the disease. So a diagnosis often comes as a shock because the man feels absolutely fine and has no suspicion that something might be wrong. Studies show that being diagnosed with prostate cancer has a significant effect on both mental health and self-rated general health.[6] But urologists and other health-care providers may not realize how bad the impact is and may instead focus on the "good news" that this is a highly curable cancer, not understanding the meaning that this has for the man and his family.

The proportion of newly diagnosed men who experience distress varies from study to study, but about 30 to 40 percent of men experience significant distress. Waiting for the results of a biopsy seems to be the most stressful time, and in one study, 65 percent of men reported stress related to the uncertainty.[7]

The extent of the distress is important, especially for the spouse who may not be sure what is normal or what needs to be done about it if it's not normal. Shock, disbelief, a feeling of "this is not happening to me," and sadness or anger are completely normal responses to a diagnosis of any kind of cancer. Anxiety and depression, however, especially if they continue for an extended period of time (more than a few days or weeks), warrant further investigation by a health-care provider and may need to be treated with medication and/or counseling.

Anxiety is characterized by excessive worry; this worry is difficult to control and is usually associated with fatigue, restlessness, irritability, difficulty concentrating, and sleep disturbance. The man may also find himself spiraling into negative thought patterns that he cannot control. Major depression is characterized by depressed mood, loss of interest and/or pleasure in daily experiences, sleeping too much or too little, feeling worthless, inability to concentrate, and thoughts of harming oneself. This is a serious mental health issue; if your spouse or partner is showing any of these signs or behaviors, he needs help immediately and should see his primary care provider as soon as possible.

What we typically see in men who are depressed or anxious is a decline in these symptoms over the next six to twelve months after the initial diagnosis. The twelve to twenty-four months after treatment is the time when recurrence is most likely, and this may cause another period of distress, accompanied by anxiety and/or depression, as uncertainty about the future is once again prevalent.

Strategies for dealing with these emotions include medication, counseling, and exercise, which can help for mild to moderate depression, as well as supportive education. Men who have experienced depression or anxiety before or who have responded to the initial diagnosis with altered mood may do well with anticipatory guidance during and after treatment when uncertainty is highest.[8] It is important to seek professional help if the man is depressed or anxious; this is not something that will go away by itself or something that you can make go away, even with your best efforts at cheering him up.

A large study from Sweden[9] found that the risk of heart attack in the week following the diagnosis of prostate cancer was almost three times higher than in men without prostate cancer. The risk of suicide in newly diagnosed men was more than eight times higher than in the general population, and younger men (less than fifty-four years old) had higher risks for both heart attack and suicide. Because this study was conducted in Sweden and not in North America, there may be cultural differences as well as differences associated with treatment options, stage of disease at diagnosis, and other factors, so the results from this study may not be applicable to men in North America. However, the importance of paying attention to the man's emotional state immediately after diagnosis is the take-home message from this study. Men may react in a very negative manner, and as the primary supports for men, partners/spouses need to listen to their intuition if they think the man is depressed or hopeless after diagnosis.

Brad and Joe have been together for almost thirty-one years. It's just been them without any family because when they told their families years ago that they were gay and in love, well, their family pretty much told them to leave and never come back. They lost so many friends in the early years of the AIDS epidemic and feel blessed that they've managed to stay healthy all these years—until last month when Joe was told that he had prostate cancer. He was devastated. Brad had never seen him like this. Joe had a tendency to be the negative one, and he made a big fuss about every little pain and cough. But he had barely gotten out of bed since he heard the news, and Brad was at a loss about what to do. He'd tried pleading and threatening and cajoling. But Joe just refused to get up. He hadn't showered in almost two weeks, and Brad had started sleeping on the couch because, well, Joe didn't smell that good, and what was the point of washing the sheets?

In desperation he called their friend Bruce who was a nurse in the ER at the big hospital downtown. Joe had told him that he couldn't breathe a word of this to anyone, but Brad just didn't know what to do. Bruce was obviously busy when Brad called his cell phone. He asked a few questions, his voice terse and clipped.

"Brad, you have to get him to his doctor. This is not a normal reaction to bad news. I'm not making a diagnosis here, okay? But this sounds like a bad depression. You have to get him some help. Bring him down here to emergency if you want, but he needs some help. You got it?"

Brad took a deep breath. He knew Bruce was right; it's what he thought he should do last week, and perhaps even the week before. Joe needed help, no matter what he said.

But how can *you* deal with your feelings of shock and distress at the diagnosis? Just as every individual is different in their response to a cancer diagnosis, so too are their spouse's/partner's responses different. And every couple copes differently too. If you need to hide your feelings to help him cope, and that is what you usually do, then that's fine. However, if you are usually the emotional one and you feel you have to act like the strong and nonemotional one, he'll notice that you are not behaving as usual, and this won't help. If you need to get your emotions out, talk to someone who can support *you*, even if your partner/spouse doesn't want to tell anyone.

People diagnosed with cancer often talk about having to support those around them instead of getting support for themselves. This can be problematic of course. But some men want to be strong; this may distract them from their own feelings and prevent them from coping effectively as discussed previously. Giving the man permission to feel and act on those feelings may be necessary, and suggesting that he doesn't have to be strong all the time may seem silly, but we have all been socialized to act in certain roles (strong man/weak woman or emotional man/calm woman) and getting permission to drop those roles, even for a brief time, can be freeing. Some men may find it so hard to admit or accept their feelings that professional help is needed. Speaking to a trained professional about his feelings after diagnosis (or at any time) can be very helpful, as the professional is at arm's length and will not judge him in any way.

Getting help for yourself in dealing with the shock of the diagnosis is important. Your coping with this can affect the man's level of distress; if you are not coping well, then he has something else to worry about. Because your distress is influenced by what you know, uncertainty and fear of the unknown and of what the future holds, and concerns about treatment, you should try and get answers to your questions about these concerns. Besides going with him to his medical appointments, ask for a referral to a social worker or patient educator at the hospital or cancer center where he is getting treatment. These professionals can help you cope effectively with your stress/distress. They can also help you find answers to many of your questions about what comes next and how best to prepare yourself for what lies ahead.

Researchers from the University of Michigan[10] conducted a study where they invited couples in which the man had prostate cancer to take part in a family-based intervention called FOCUS. The intervention provided information and education about five key areas: family involvement, optimistic attitude, coping effectiveness, uncertainty reduction, and symptom management. The group who took part in these sessions was then compared to another group of prostate cancer patients and spouses. Not surprisingly, the spouses of the men in the intervention group did much better than the other spouses who had not received the education sessions, and they also did better than the patients! These spouses had more confidence in their ability to care for and support the man, experienced less uncertainty about the illness, and felt less hopeless. The spouses also experienced better personal quality of life as a result of being encouraged to deal with their own health issues and eat well and get some exercise. Couples who participated in the educational sessions also improved their communication about the disease.

DON'T ASK, DON'T TELL

Men differ in whom they tell about the diagnosis, when they talk about it, and how much they disclose. In one study,[11] men stated that they needed to manage the impact of the diagnosis, and they did it in five ways. First they needed to deal with the practicalities of having cancer, and this could involve setting up appointments with doctors and making a treatment decision. They also felt the need to prevent the illness from interfering with daily life and so went about their usual routines. Third, they wanted to keep relationships working and so maintained contact with their usual friends and family members. An important part of managing the impact of the illness was managing their feelings and controlling their expression of emotion. And finally, the men in this study talked about making sense of it all, figuring out what this meant for their overall way of being in the world and how to live after prostate cancer.

───── ∽∾∾∽ ─────

In the three months since Sam had received his diagnosis of prostate cancer, his wife Carla had been having a hard time. He had told her that she was not to tell anyone *about it, and the look on his face allowed no argument. He'd always been the one to make the rules in their marriage, and she had usually obeyed. He had a fierce temper and for all the years of their marriage, forty-five at their last anniversary, she and their children had been careful not to cause him to lose it. But it was so hard for her to deal with this. He didn't say much about what the doctors told him; she wasn't sure he'd even gone back to see the doctor. He'd just told her about it one evening after dinner and warned her not to speak about it to any of her "hen friends," as he described the women from her church group.*

She'd prayed about it, and once she almost told their pastor about it, but the fear of Sam's reaction made her hold her tongue. She wasn't sleeping properly, and her nerves felt like the edge of her knife that she used every day to make salad. She didn't know what to expect—was he going to die?—and he refused to talk about it. So she watched him and waited, but for what? For him to get sick, or to ask for help? She worried about him because he didn't go to church and he didn't lead a good life in her view. How could he bear this without the help of anyone? She had so many questions and no answers, and she felt so alone for the first time in her life.

Some men need time to let things settle, to get used to the idea of having cancer before they want to tell others or even talk to their spouse or partner about anything. Other men feel that there are certain people that they have to tell; they have a sense of obligation that their boss needs to know, or their close friends, or perhaps even just some of their siblings. They may avoid telling an elderly parent, or friends or relatives who have their own health issues. This ability to disclose may in part be based on what the man expects the response will be, or how stigmatizing he thinks the disease is. Because prostate cancer affects sexuality, there may be a perception that the disease is embarrassing or makes him less of a man. This negative attribution may cause him to avoid telling anyone, or at least to minimize who will know. This can affect you directly; you may want to seek support for yourself, or you may want to garner support for him as an individual and for both of you as a couple. Often disclosure is something that is negotiated over time—you tell just a very few of your closest friends at first, but as he gets used to the idea and manages the illness, you start to tell more and more of your friends and family.

Men may talk to strangers about their diagnosis before they are ready to talk to their close friends. This is not strange, particularly if the men they are talking to have gone through the experience. Some men are very open about their cancer at support group meetings but may want you to keep it a secret from your children. The reason for this is that, first, the other men at the support group are strangers and are, in his mind, less likely to judge him. Second, they have gone through what he is going through and can provide him with information to help him adjust to the news and figure out what to do, and in addition they are proof that there is life after cancer.

Other men talk about their diagnosis widely. They may see an altruistic purpose to disclosure and feel the need to impress upon their friends and coworkers that they too need to be tested. You may not feel the same way; it may be that *you* want to keep it quiet, for a short or even a long while. But you have to go with what he wants in this instance, because *he* is the one with the cancer. Yes, it has a profound effect on you and your life together, but ultimately it is his cancer and he can tell or not tell. Some men use humor as a way of dealing with the diagnosis. This may be upsetting to you, because you don't see anything funny about the situation. Humor is often used to deal with difficult situations, and this may be the only way that he can talk about it. Humor is often used to deflect others from making fun of oneself, so men may choose to joke about the possibility of urinary leakage or erectile difficulties rather than imagining other men making jokes at their expense first.

Carl had always been the life and soul of any party. People often said he should be on TV with his own show, he was so funny. And he dealt with his prostate cancer the same way. His wife June mostly went along with it—there wasn't much she could do about his big personality anyway. And since he'd known about the cancer, he'd insisted that every second Wednesday night they go to the support group meeting at the clinic near their home.

Carl had found a new audience for his jokes, but this time the jokes were uncomfortable for June. He joked about wearing diapers and he joked about sex, and she just cringed. The other men at the support group seemed to enjoy his jokes and off-color comments; but she could see that the other wives were uncomfortable, and when they broke for coffee, none of the other women approached her. Carl had a group of men around him as he continued to tell his "funny" stories, but she stood alone, trying to act like she didn't care, but she really did. He was making a fool of himself in her eyes, and by association, she looked foolish too.

She tried talking to him in the car after the last meeting.

"Oh honey, you're just being silly," he said with a big grin on his face. "The guys love it! Hey, like I always say, if you can't laugh at yourself you may as well be dead!"

At the word "dead," June started to cry. She'd tried to hide her tears from him until now, but she couldn't help herself.

"Honey, what's the matter? Why are you crying?"

June could barely get the words out: "Why am I crying? You have to ask? I'm crying because my husband has cancer and he thinks it's a joke! I'm crying because

I don't want to lose you and you don't seem to care! That's why I'm crying, Carl. Because I'm scared and I'm sad, and all you do is make stupid jokes!"

There was silence in the car, just the sound of the air rushing past the window that was open on the driver's side. Carl stared straight ahead and June sniffed. When she sneaked a look at his face it was slack. For once he was not smiling or making a joke. He looked like he'd been hit in the face.

And then there are the men who want their spouse or partner to do the disclosing for them. They encourage you to tell everyone you feel needs to know, and in that way they don't have to say the words "I have cancer" over and over again. They avoid any uncomfortable moments when the recipient of the news looks shocked or doesn't know what to say. In some ways, this avoids emotional interactions with those they love. By having you tell your children or close friends and family members, the man is not exposed to their pain and sorrow and can avoid feeling those emotions himself.

Like anything else in the cancer journey, when it comes to telling others about the diagnosis, there is no perfect way to do it. Take your lead from him, but don't be afraid to voice your opinion. As difficult as this is for him, you are affected too, and you have a right to express yourself and make your feelings known. But ultimately this is his cancer, and, in the beginning at least, you have to take your lead from him. But over time things will change, and he will be more likely to talk about it with those who are important to him, starting with you.

WHAT COMES NEXT . . .

It's better for the couple to take some time after the diagnosis before deciding on what treatment the man wants to have. Many men just want to get it over with and opt for whatever the physician says he should do. If the physician is a surgeon, the recommendation is usually surgery. If the physician is a radiation oncologist, the recommendation is usually some form of radiation. That makes sense. But it may not make sense for the man, and even though he wants to get it done and dealt with, taking some time to make a treatment decision after consideration of all the side effects is a better idea. It's important that you fully understand what the options are and, just as important, what the side effects of the various treatments are. You'll read more about this in upcoming chapters.

· 3 ·

Is This the Right Doctor?

Choosing a Doctor and Treatment

*N*ow that you know all about the diagnosis, what do you do next? Should the recommended treatment be accepted, or should you explore other options? What about getting a second or third opinion? And what do you need to think about when weighing all the options?

Once a man learns of his diagnosis, things will never be the same for either him or you. An individual once called it "being in Cancerland," a world where uncertainty rules and nothing is the same as it was before. One of the unique things about prostate cancer is that most men are asked to decide what treatment they want. This is very different from almost every other kind of cancer, where treatment protocols are clear and the patient has the treatment that is recommended.

    In part because prostate cancer is usually diagnosed at an early stage, any of the established treatments are likely to be effective in curing the cancer. In addition, prostate cancer tends to be a slow-growing cancer, so most men die of something other than the cancer. This results in a great deal of ambiguity for the man and his partner/spouse, making the process of deciding on a treatment stressful and difficult. One of the positive things about prostate cancer, if one can say that any cancer has a positive side, is that because it is usually slow growing, you have time to learn more about the disease and its treatments, and time to make a treatment decision. Nothing has to happen in a hurry, even though in your heart you may feel that action needs to be taken immediately. Many men, and sometimes their partners too, want immediate treatment—the same day as they learn about the diagnosis in some cases! Some doctors also encourage their patients to make a treatment decision quickly, thinking that having treatment immediately will reduce their stress.

This is not necessary and can actually cause more problems than it solves. Decision making about prostate cancer treatment is often described as a quality-of-life decision, and making decisions that will affect the man's quality of life, and yours by association, deserves some time and careful thought.

For men with localized prostate cancer, the choice is between surgery, different forms of radiation, or some newer, experimental treatments. It is really a decision about quality of life, because all of the treatments have side effects that will affect him for the rest of his (hopefully) long life. In the process of decision making, there is a new language to be learned, side effects are seen as being weighed against life-and-death considerations, and these things all happen at a time when it is difficult to think clearly and logically. In the following chapters you will read about the various treatments in detail, but this chapter describes the process of making a decision about treatment. It is an important one for you to read as the major support person for the man with prostate cancer.

PHYSICIAN FACTORS

The beginning of the cancer journey for most men with prostate cancer begins with the disclosure of the diagnosis by a physician. Depending on the type of specialist, urologist versus radiation oncologist, a recommendation for treatment may be made by this physician. This can be highly influential in the eventual decision the man makes, and some men will accept this recommendation and not seek further information or another opinion. In one study, urologists (who are surgeons) overwhelmingly recommended surgery for their prostate cancer patients; 93 percent stated that this was the preferred treatment. Seventy-two percent of radiation oncologists stated that radiation therapy and surgery were equivalent in their potential to treat prostate cancer, but both types of specialists were much more likely to recommend the treatment they provided than any other form of treatment.[1]

How the diagnosis is communicated, and further communication about the various treatment options, is very important not only for the treatment choice that the man makes, but also for his comfort and trust after treatment when quality-of-life side effects come to the fore. Times have changed, and it is generally accepted that patients have the right to accept or refuse treatment, seek information, and play an active role in treatment decision making. Older men and older physicians may see this differently however!

In the past, physicians often did take a paternalistic approach to providing information to patients. "The doctor knows best" was the dominant attitude, and most patients, regardless of age, accepted this. The physician in most instances was better educated, held more power, and was used to telling patients what to do. In response, patients listened and obeyed and didn't question the authority, knowledge, and experience of the physician. But things are different today; patients have greater access to the specialized knowledge held by health-care providers through the Internet and media in general. There is also a loosening of the boundaries between experts and laypeople, and so the authority of physicians is not as entrenched as it was decades ago.

An interesting study was conducted some years ago in which urologists were asked what questions they thought should be addressed with patients who have prostate cancer.[2] The questions identified as being important to be answered were the rates of incontinence after surgery (identified as important by 76 percent of physician respondents), cure rates (74 percent), and erectile difficulties after surgery (73 percent). The questions identified as being those to avoid included searching for the best medical center (29 percent) and the number of prostate cancer patients cured by the physician (16 percent). You can see from this what makes doctors uncomfortable!

Sam is sixty-eight years old and for the past six months has been having more and more problems with his "waterworks." He gets up to pass urine at least five times a night, and this is disturbing his wife Sylvia. They are both tired and grumpy, and they've started to fight a lot more. So Sylvia didn't go with Sam to a couple of doctor's appointments, and she is shocked when he comes home one day, his face white and his voice trembling.

"I have to have surgery! Syl, I have cancer! How did this happen?"

Sylvia tries to keep calm, but it feels like every cell in her body is screaming.

"What do you mean, Sam? Surgery? Cancer? Sit down and start at the beginning."

Sam tells her everything—his family doctor sent him to a specialist and he had a biopsy (Sylvia can't begin to figure out how he kept this from her), and today the specialist told him he had cancer and he needed surgery. Sylvia listens, asks a few questions, and then picks up the phone to call their son Bruce, who's a dentist in Miami. He has lots of friends in the medical business, and he'll know what to do. Bruce is indeed helpful; his father-in-law had prostate cancer two years before, and he remembers the process he went through before having treatment.

"Tell Dad that he doesn't necessarily have to have surgery. And give me the name of this doctor he saw; I'm going to call him and get some details. And then I'm going to fly home next weekend and help you sort this out. Just tell Dad not to agree to anything before we've talked!"

Sylvia smiled for the first time—Bruce still thought of Chicago as "home" even though he hadn't lived here for almost ten years! And he was going to help them through this! She felt better already.

———— ∞∞∞ ————

The physician should give the man enough information so that he can make a decision that is right for him, and that information must be tailored to the patient's preference for receiving medical information. This is not as easy as it sounds! Being able to provide the patient with information at the right level and with the preferred amount of detail while at the same time figuring out how much the patient wants to participate in decision making is a complex process. The physician also needs to explain the rationale for any treatment recommendations he or she makes to the patient. This is a lot of information, usually is exchanged in a brief visit, and it may be a tall order to carry out properly and to the satisfaction of either or both the physician and the patient, not to mention the man's partner or spouse. Not all physicians are expert communicators and educators, and this takes time, something that is often in short supply in a busy practice. You can ask to make another appointment to come back and discuss things again and ask more questions. As you read in the previous chapter, it is not unusual to hear very little after the words "You have cancer" are spoken. So if you feel that you are overwhelmed with the information being given, take a breath and ask if you can come back another time to talk some more. And before that visit, make sure that you do some searching of your own so that both of you are better informed and able to ask important questions.

Physicians should also consider what they know about the patient's health and any existing problems likely to be affected by the treatments offered. However this does not always happen. In a study of almost five hundred men with prostate cancer, 89 percent reported that they had existing urinary, bowel, or sexual problems, but this appeared to be ignored by the physicians treating them. More than a third of these men received treatments that worsened their existing problems, and active surveillance, the treatment option with the least side effects in these areas, was very infrequently offered.[3] This is an important area where you can act as an advocate for your spouse or partner. He may be reluctant to admit to problems, or he may not be asked about existing problems. Many people don't bring up issues if not specifically asked about them, and you can play a vital role in bringing any problems to the physician's attention.

Not all men will stay throughout the treatment with the physician who made the diagnosis; finding the right fit between the treating physician and the man is important, although not all patients are aware that they can seek another opinion or change physicians. Of course, if you live in a smaller city or one that is remote, the choices may be limited. The man may not feel comfortable with the communication style of the physician or with the level and amount of information provided. Some men will seek advice from others who have had prostate cancer and will seek treatment from the physician recommended by other survivors. It may be difficult for the man to assess the competency of the suggested physician objectively, but a heartfelt endorsement from one or more cancer survivors may be enough to help him make up his mind, even if the recommended physician has less than perfect bedside manner or poor communication skills.

Surgery volume or how many procedures the physician has performed is often suggested as a way of assessing the competence of the surgeon. It is well established that the greater the number of surgeries the surgeon has performed, the better the outcomes for the patients. However one study suggests that even in surgeons who do many operations, surgical technique is also an important factor, so doing a lot of operations using bad technique does not have the same outcomes as doing many surgeries with good technique.[4]

Many patient education booklets and websites have a list of questions that they suggest be asked of any physician seen as part of the decision-making process. These often include questions such as the following:

- What treatment, or treatments, do you recommend for me/my spouse or partner?
- How does the rate of side effects we have read about on the Web compare to the rate of side effects in your practice?
- How likely is my/his cancer to come back in the next five or ten years?
- How frequently will I/he have to see a doctor after being treated?
- Will I/he have to have more tests?
- Who can we talk with about problems holding urine or having erections after treatment?
- Where can he find a support group?
- Does his age, or current health, indicate any treatment that is better for him? (adapted from the Prostate Cancer Decision website: http://www.prostatecancerdecision.org)

It is very important that the physician spend enough time with the man and his partner/spouse, and that your questions be answered to your satisfaction. Curt and flippant answers are indicative of someone who is not that interested in the patient and his support person and may suggest how future problems and queries will be dealt with. Using medical terms that the patient and partner don't understand is not helpful and may prevent further questions or requests for clarification. No one likes to feel stupid, and having a doctor talk way over your head is not conducive to learning and understanding about something that will affect both of you for the rest of your lives. Physicians often present information about the treatment options and side effects or complications in the form of statistics or numbers. They often use population statistics where a number or proportion is drawn from studies in which large numbers of men have been studied to explain something that the patient wants to understand from an individual or personal perspective. It is often difficult to understand these statistics and their meaning for one's own situation.[5] It is not unreasonable to ask for a translation of statistics or numbers that are confusing into real language. Many people receive information but then interpret it incorrectly; surgery for prostate cancer is often seen by patients and family as a guarantee of a cure, which it is not. And many men decide on a treatment after seeing the urologist just once.

Hank was diagnosed with prostate cancer two months ago. He still doesn't know what treatment he wants, and his longtime girlfriend, Margot, is getting frustrated with him. They usually take their trailer down to Phoenix in the winter, and September is fast approaching. She wants him to make a decision so that she can start making plans for their trip. But Hank needs more time.

He remembers that a friend of a friend had prostate cancer last year and after some digging around, he gets his phone number and they meet for coffee the following day. Dan is the guy's name. He's a retired police officer who keeps his silver hair short and his shoulders back. He listens as Hank talks about his concerns.

"I know it makes sense to just get the damn thing out and then I never have to think about it again. But there's just something about going under the knife that makes me feel sick, you know? The doctor I saw is very confident that he can get it all, and he's very busy, which means he's good, right? But still, I'm not sure."

Dan clears his throat before replying.

"Now, everyone is different, mind, but I was just like you. I also thought that if I had surgery it would be taken care of. And it was, for a while. I didn't realize that after the surgery you still have to watch things, and my last two PSA readings haven't been that good."

He didn't make eye contact with Hank as he continued, his deep voice a little tighter and higher.

"Anyway, they think that they didn't get it all after all that. So now I have to have radiation, and I could have just had that in the first place. I listened to the guy too—very slick he was in his fancy office in a high-rise downtown—and I didn't

ask too many questions because I don't think I wanted to think too much about it. Just get it out and then I'd be done. But I'm not done, not at all."

It was now Hank's turn to clear his throat. What do you say to a guy after hearing that?

It has been shown that men evaluate the information they receive at diagnosis not only in terms of what they are told, but also how they are told. Warmth and empathy from the physician are important to men and influence how they understand the information provided to them.[6] Other experts[7] agree that the essential strategies for quality decision making are providing clear explanations, checking that the patient understands what he has been told, asking what the patient's values are, assessing his concerns and needs, finding common ground and reaching agreement on the treatment plan, and establishing an acceptable follow-up plan. Is this what you and your partner/spouse experienced in the doctor's office?

Physicians sometimes use tools that help them predict how a man's cancer may behave in terms of coming back or spreading in his body. These tools (called nomograms) are thought to be more accurate than physicians' clinical judgment. There are many different nomograms available, and many physicians have them on their smart phones and can input the results of tests for a specific man and see what the probability is of spread, progression, or survival. The results are usually given in percentages (e.g., there is a less than 25 percent chance that the cancer has spread to the lymph nodes) and can be difficult to understand.[8]

Physicians often provide written information in the form of books or pamphlets. These are often provided by pharmaceutical or industry representatives and may contain information about a specific drug or piece of equipment used by the physician. While these are usually of high printing quality, the information presented may be biased in favor of the medication or equipment made by the company; it can be difficult to identify this bias, so you may be misinformed or not have balanced information from reading that particular publication. Some printed materials don't provide comprehensive content; one study found that of the pamphlets they examined, at least one treatment option was left out in six of the nine studied (usually the option of active surveillance), and the stated risks of side effects were vague and in some cases absent entirely.[9]

Some physicians employ nurses or other allied health professionals to assist them in providing information to patients as part of the treatment decision-making process; this is often described as consultation planning.[10]

This process is intended to help the patient be a more active participant in treatment decision making, and when used with decision aids it has been found to improve decision quality and increase patient satisfaction. This may be the best solution as, unlike reading a book or pamphlet or visiting a website, there is the opportunity to ask questions and express thoughts and opinions. Some physicians use decision aids to assist patients, and these are discussed in the section below.

Decision Aids

Patient decision aids are tools that provide information about the risks and benefits of specific treatments, explain medical conditions, and present ways for the reader to clarify personal values. Most are self-administered and are available in paper format, on DVDs or videos, or as computer software. They are often available on cancer agency or disease-specific websites.

Decision aids have been found to improve knowledge and encourage more active patient involvement in decision making (something that many men say they want), and they may also decrease anxiety and distress.[11] They also help you to understand the risks and benefits of various treatment options and can reduce the difficulty of making a decision. Physicians support their use for the most part, stating that patients are more prepared for a discussion after using a decision aid and are better able to state what their preferences are, and such aids help patients talk about treatment options with medical practitioners and family members. However, these aids appear to influence patient choice, which may not please all physicians; in one study, 60 percent of those men who used a decision aid chose a different treatment than the surgeon originally recommended. This may be a result of the patient learning new information about alternative treatments or receiving more information about side effects.

Bill was referred to a cancer center in another town after he was diagnosed with prostate cancer. His family nurse practitioner explained that there were a lot of specialists there, and he would get good care. He wasn't sure that he would be any better off there than with Doc Brown, the local urologist, and he wasn't that keen on driving for three hours to get there, but his wife Marcy persuaded him to go.

To his surprise, when he got there he didn't see a doctor but instead someone who called herself a "clinical nurse specialist." This woman explained that her role was to help patients and their partners come to a treatment decision that was right for them and their life together. He looked at Marcy over the table, and she just lifted her eyebrows at him and smiled. So he sat back and listened. Sandy—that was her name—went over the results of his PSA test and biopsy results. Marcy was paying a lot of attention to this, making notes in her neat teacher's handwriting, and nodding as Sandy explained what all of it meant.

Then Sandy started talking about the various treatments, and Bill was now listening intently. She told them much more than the urologist in his hometown had told them. She went on about urine leakage, and she even talked about erections! Bill was a bit shocked at that, but Marcy seemed to know all about it. She'd been searching on the Internet for information ever since he learned about the cancer, but he didn't really want to know all the details of what she'd found. Doc Brown had said surgery was the best treatment for him, and he was the expert after all. But as he listened, he started to think about things, and he wasn't at all sure that he wanted to have surgery anymore. Sandy said that with his kind of cancer, he could have a special kind of radiation—"seeds" she called it—and that was sounding much better than being cut open. Marcy just smiled reassuringly at him and continued to write in her little notebook. Boy, he had a lot to think about!

Another form of decision aid is question prompt sheets. These contain a set of questions that have been found to be helpful to patients in accessing information that enables them to make treatment decisions. The questions may be similar to those listed above from the Prostate Cancer Decision website. They usually contain specific questions about grade and stage of prostate cancer in addition to questions about cure rates, side effects, and so forth. Studies show that these prompt sheets lead patients to ask more questions. Patients state that their information needs are better met, but there is no indication that their understanding increased or that their anxiety about the cancer was decreased at all. It has also been shown that these prompt sheets help patients to recall information, but only if the physician approves of using them and pays attention to the questions the patient asks.[12]

Decision aids are available from the following websites:

- Foundation for Informed Medical Decision Making (www.fimdm.org)
- Healthwise (www.healthwise.org)
- Mayo Clinic (www.mayoclinic.org)

PATIENT FACTORS

Choosing a treatment for prostate cancer is a complex process for any man. Consideration must be given to the extent and aggressiveness of the cancer, as well as to the health of the man himself and any medical conditions he has. Personal preferences for treatment and attitudes toward the different options for treatment must also be taken into account. Men also consider the experience of family and friends who have had cancer as well as factors such as time away from work and costs of treatment. In addition, men must think about the potential for side effects and anticipate what side effects they are prepared to live with and which would be unacceptable to them. This is a tall order and often occurs at a time when the man is in crisis after hearing the diagnosis and his levels of uncertainty are very high.

The results of a study using in-depth interviews with prostate cancer patients identified some interesting factors that men may take into consideration when making a decision about treatment.[13] Men described how the uncertainty of experts (the various physicians they saw) and the lack of agreement on the best treatment increased their own uncertainty. Most of us desire certainty in our lives, and for the most part we think we have such certainty, until something like cancer happens, which is never in our life plan! In this study, some men found the statistics and probabilities that the doctor presented to them to be useful. A small number of men in this study chose active surveillance (sometimes called "watchful waiting" and addressed in chapter 4 of this book) because this was one treatment that was reversible, while all the others were permanent. The men in this study also wanted to take their time making a decision because they thought that they could find more information if they did not rush into things. Still others wanted to make a decision quickly and "get it over with."

Another study highlighted the factors that men consider when making a decision about treatment.[14] For some men and their partners, getting rid of the cancer is the primary consideration, and they are prepared to deal with the consequences of that in the future. For other men, their primary concern is quality of life, and they consider the side effects of the various treatment options in light of the specific side effects. Urinary incontinence appears to be of greater importance than sexual difficulties for men and their partners. This topic will be covered in greater detail in subsequent chapters.

Physician recommendation is another important factor for some men, and in one study it was the strongest predictor of treatment choice.[15] Despite the bias that has been shown to occur, as described earlier in this chapter, many men regard the opinion of their physician as being very important in their decision. This may be because the physician is seen as the technical expert who is best able to guide the man or because the physician is seen as having provided information to the man, even though the information may be limited and biased and the man may not be aware of this. In one study, 59 percent of men had not considered any treatment other than surgery, and the opinion of friends was the most important factor in their decision.[16]

This is another area where the presence of a spouse or partner can be priceless. You are likely to seek out additional information, and you can provide a necessary balance if your partner/spouse appears to be accepting advice without much thought or critique. You may be the one who is assigned to do the reading and the searching for more information because you have always done this, and he may not read anything at all, which can be frustrating given that it is his body and his life. Some men say that they feel pressure from their spouse and other family members to treat the cancer aggressively; it is natural to want the man you all love to live as long as possible even with diminished quality of life. But he may not agree with this and may make a decision that you don't like or agree with. Studies indicate that in the end, most spouses believe that the final decision should be his, despite your feelings about what you think is right or better for him.

It is important that the man play an active role in treatment decision making because this has been shown to limit the amount of regret the man may experience after he has had the treatment.[17] For some men who don't take the time to explore their options or who don't learn more about the side effects of treatment, living with these side effects can lead to regret about having that treatment. This is called "decisional regret" and can have a negative effect on coping for many years after treatment. Being an active participant in decision making does not mean that the man makes the decision alone; most men want their physicians to be involved in guiding them toward a decision. They want their spouse/partner to be part of the decision too; we will talk more about the role of the spouse/partner later in this chapter.

Jim was an Iraq war veteran—the first Iraq war that is—and his whole life had been spent making decisions quickly and decisively. That was the way he lived his life; he thought about things in an analytic and rational way and then decided what to do. And in his family, his word was final. He had grown up in an army family, and back then, things were really strict. He liked his life to be ordered and orderly, and his wife Sue and his two sons, Brent and Jim Jr., for the most part went along with that.

Being diagnosed with prostate cancer threw him for a loop. This was not what he had planned! He went to the VA clinic for all his medical needs, and he had faith in the doctors and nurses there. They'd taken good care of him when he came back from Iraq with some weird lung problem, and he was sure that they'd take good care of him now too.

Sue wanted to learn more about the treatments, and she wanted to tell Jim all about it, but he wasn't interested. The medical staff were the experts; they knew what was best, he told her, and that was how he was going to handle things. Sue knew better than to argue with him when he'd made up his mind, so she didn't talk about what she had found out on the Internet anymore. She was scared about what she had read, scared about how Jim would be if he couldn't control his bladder; but he didn't want to talk about it, and there was nothing she could do about that. So she worried and she waited until the day of his surgery. They would just have to deal with the fallout when it happened.

Personality factors also play a role. Men who make decisions quickly in other parts of their lives may be more inclined to make a quick decision in this situation, perhaps to their detriment if they are not fully informed about the side effects of the particular treatment they have chosen. Men who are natural pessimists have been shown to have more difficulty with treatment decision making than their optimistic counterparts.[18] This may be because they have lower self-confidence in their ability to make a decision. Most of us know the personality of our partner as well as we know our own, and you can be of great help if you know that the man you love is a pessimist; he may need additional support around his ability to choose what is right for him and not second-guess himself.

The amount and quality of information that the man accesses in order to make a treatment decision varies widely. Younger men, and those with higher education and income, tend to seek out additional information about prostate cancer and its treatment beyond what they are told by their physician.[19] Outside of the physician, 76 percent of men report using pamphlets and videos, other health-care providers (71 percent), friends with prostate cancer (67 percent), and the Internet (58 percent). The Internet provided men with the most treatment options to consider.[20] People who use the Internet to access information have been found to be more active in treatment decision making than those who don't, and education level did not have any effect, so Internet use is seen to be useful for patients.[21]

While some men seek a second opinion, many find that multiple treatment recommendations just confuse things more. Others find that multiple opinions reduce bias for them and provide them with useful information to make a decision.[22] Some men may not understand the purpose of getting a second opinion; they may think it is merely to confirm what they have already heard. A second opinion from the same kind of specialist may not be helpful in the context of prostate cancer, given what you have read in this chapter about specialists recommending their own type of treatment. Seeing a radiation oncologist after seeing a urologist and vice versa may be of more use in terms of information gathering and reducing bias.

A treatment decision is also sometimes made in the heat of the moment and may be heavily influenced by fear, uncertainty, and the desire to do something quickly. Misconceptions about the various treatment options are common (for example, that surgical removal of the prostate is 100 percent effective in treating the cancer). Men also make decisions based on the experience of others with the same cancer, even if the stage and extent of the other man's cancer are very different. Some men have beliefs about cancer or the treatment that fly in the face of science, but these are very important in their decision-making process. An example of this is those who believe that if you cut near cancer, the cancer will spread. There is no factual basis for this, but it is a strong belief. Others believe that radiation will cause cancer somewhere else in the body or that it is mysterious and because you can't see its effect, it is less successful.

Brad is relatively young to have been diagnosed with prostate cancer. At forty-six years of age, he'd been having his PSA measured because his dad had prostate cancer in his sixties and his brother had been diagnosed a year earlier. He always thought he would get it one day, just not in his forties, but he got used to the idea quite quickly and seemed calm despite the news.

The only problem was when he told his urologist that he didn't want to have surgery.

"What do you mean?" the urologist seemed shocked. "This is the best treatment for a man at your age. It gives you the best chance of cure, and because you're young, you'll just bounce back. In two or three months you won't even feel like you've had surgery!"

"I want to have the seed implant," Brad explained to the doctor, whose face was red and whose arms were crossed over his chest, making him look like his old high school principal. "I know what my dad went through after his surgery, and I don't want that to happen to me. And my brother hasn't had an erection in a year, and they told him he'd be as good as he was before! So don't try and persuade me about anything! I want to see the radiation doc, and I want to see him soon!"

The urologist shook his head and pulled out a form and began to tick the boxes. If Brad wanted a different treatment, it was his choice, even if the doctor thought it was the wrong choice. Some men are just like that.

The good news is that despite experiencing difficulty and distress while making a treatment decision (almost half of all men in one study), most men had no regrets with the decision they eventually made.[23] This may in part be a coping mechanism whereby the man tries to justify his choice of treatment, despite suffering from a variety of side effects. Treatment regret does occur, though, usually among a minority of men, and it is most likely to occur six months to a year after treatment.[24] This is a time when the reality of ongoing problems with side effects sinks in and the man has to accept that they are not short term. The support of the partner/spouse is very important for these men but may be challenging if you thought he should have made a different decision at the outset.

PARTNER FACTORS

Most of this chapter has been written about what the man has to think about and do in the process of making a treatment choice. And now you are reading a section on what the partner can/should/must do. This division is somewhat false because prostate cancer is a couple's disease. One could say that about any disease, more or less. But the research shows over and over that the partner of the man with prostate cancer is usually intimately involved in all stages of the disease, as well as many years after treatment is over and the man is cured of his disease or when he faces the terminal stages of it.

Being partnered is important for health generally, and it's even more important when the man faces cancer. Married men are more likely to choose a definitive treatment (surgery or radiation) than are their single counterparts.[25] There has been no research on men who are not married but are living in long-term relationships; the assumption might be made that it is not marital status but rather partner status that is important. We also know that spouses/partners often take the lead in seeking out information. They also appear to place more importance on cure than the man does; he may consider side effects more in his treatment decision making.[26] However, spouses repeatedly say that ultimately it is the man's choice as he has to live with the consequences of the treatment, so the partner's role is seen as being more supportive and encouraging. In one study, 54 percent of men wanted to share the decision making with their partner, and about the same percentage of partners wanted to play a collaborative role in the treatment the man chose. But 42 percent of the partners did not want to play an active role and preferred to be passive.[27]

Studies have identified repeatedly that the information needs of both the men and their partners are high at the time of diagnosis and are often not met by health-care providers. So the spouse or partner seeks out that information and tries to make sense of it at a time when it is difficult to process complicated facts and information because of the distress related to the man's new diagnosis.[28] Seeking out information can be both empowering and overwhelming, the end result of which may be more uncertainty and an inability to move forward and make a decision.[29] It is not uncommon for the spouse/partner to read widely and get frustrated when the man seems to not be interested in reading the same material. Individual preferences for involvement in decision making vary widely, as do assumptions of who should be making the decision. The partner may assume that he/she has a greater role to play because of the amount of information he/she has gathered and read. But the man may reject that notion and ask his specialist to tell him what to do.

Men and their partners also see things differently; you may need help in accepting this, as these perceptions may last for many years after diagnosis and can be a source of frustration and conflict for the couple. For example, the man may place greater importance on sexual functioning than his partner, who would trade sex for his life any day. While cancer certainly changes the world for the man with prostate cancer and his partner, it does not fundamentally change the way the couple acts or the norms of their relationship. Pessimists and optimists deal with cancer much like they deal with anything else in life, and you can't expect an optimist to suddenly become less hopeful even if you don't feel that much hope. And a pessimist is going to approach a diagnosis of cancer with an attitude of doom and gloom no matter what you say.

Lois and Chuck had a fight in the doctor's office, right in front of him! They often didn't see eye to eye, but they usually kept their differences private. But this time Lois couldn't hold her tongue.

"What do you mean you don't want to have treatment for this cancer? Are you crazy? Or is this some kind of sick joke? Who cares about sex at a time like this? I just can't believe you're thinking like this!"

"Butt out, Lois! This is my body you're talking about!"

"But this is our marriage! Do you honestly think that I care more about your damn penis than I do about your life?"

Lois was shaking in anger, and she felt her eyes fill up with tears. She'd shed more than a few tears in the week since they'd found out about the prostate cancer. But these were tears of anger and frustration and loss of control. The doctor tried to interrupt, but Lois and Chuck seemed to have forgotten that he was even in the room.

"It's not about you, Lois! For once in your life can you just keep out of things? For me it is about my damn penis, as you so described it. I'm not prepared to live out my life with a limp . . ."

"Don't you dare say it, Chuck! Don't you dare! I've had enough of this and enough of you! Can't you think about your kids and grandkids if you don't want to

think about me? I'm sorry, doctor, but I can't be a part of this. Let him do what he wants! I can't listen to another word!"

    And she left the room, her coat still on the chair back. Chuck just sighed and the doctor sighed, and they sat in silence for a moment. And then Chuck started asking questions.

—∞∞∞—

Men may not share their feelings at this time, and to the partner, this can feel like rejection or alienation. Some men may go alone to the appointment where the results of the biopsy are disclosed, hear the diagnosis of prostate cancer, and come home unable to get the words out. The partner knows that something is going on; the man looks upset and may be irritable or withdrawn, but the partner has no idea of the gravity of the situation.

    You will hear over and over in the chapters of this book about the importance of you attending all medical appointments, and that includes visits to allied health professionals like physiotherapists too. There is a simple explanation for this: four ears are better than two. It allows you to hear information firsthand and improves recall for both of you. And sharing this challenge allows for something called posttraumatic growth, a positive emotional outcome after facing something very challenging. Posttraumatic growth can be experienced as greater closeness between partners, enhanced personal relationships with family and friends, and more satisfactory relationship quality.[30] Couples also make sense of the cancer over time, and for some, cancer is seen as a "good cancer" because survival rates are so high and most men die with the disease rather than from it.[31]

WHAT COMES NEXT . . .

There's a lot to learn about the different kinds of treatment, and every day in the media you can read about a new and innovative treatment that is cutting edge. But is it really? How does it compare with treatments that are well established and have been used by hundreds of thousands of men for several decades? In the following chapters you will read about the different kinds of treatments for prostate cancer, from active surveillance and surgery to radiation and then to some newer treatments that are not as well accepted. You will learn about the pros and cons of each, the effectiveness and side effects of the treatment, and all of this should help you become more informed and better able to support and help the man you love make a decision that is right for him, and hopefully you too, in the context of your relationship.

Waiting It Out

Active Surveillance

$\mathscr{T}$here are some men who don't need treatment for prostate cancer immediately, if at all, and they can be followed closely for many years without any
definitive treatment being necessary. Active surveillance is increasingly being
offered to men as a way of delaying or avoiding treatment while preserving
quality of life.

Increasingly, physicians are realizing that many men with prostate cancer are
being overtreated. What does this mean? Basically, there is recognition that
not all men diagnosed with prostate cancer need active treatment in the form
of surgery or radiation or even one of the newer and experimental treatments.
But how can these experts allow men to go without treatment? A key to
understanding this lies in understanding the concept of delayed or deferred
treatment, something that is becoming more widely used in the management
of low-risk prostate cancer.

Discussing deferred or delayed treatment for prostate cancer requires
both a history lesson as well as a crash course in prostate cancer clinical markers. An explanation of the language used to describe prostate cancer and its
treatment is also necessary. To go over the history, please refer back to chapter 1. That chapter describes the PSA test, the clinical stage of the cancer,
and the Gleason score, the only method we have at the present time to predict
how prostate cancer may act in an individual man.

Now for the language lesson: this may seem a little silly, but what we
call this treatment strategy is confusing and can make a great deal of difference in what the patient and his partner/spouse understand. The terms
used (such as "delayed/deferred treatment," "conservative management,"
"active surveillance," and "watchful waiting") are important, as they too

reflect some of the history of prostate cancer treatment. In addition, health-care providers may use one of the terms but really mean something else. Traditionally, not offering a man with prostate cancer curative treatment (surgery or radiation therapy) was referred to as "watchful waiting." Essentially, health-care providers watched the man and waited for signs of disease progression and spread outside of the prostate gland. At that point, the man was usually given palliative (that is, noncurative) treatment in the form of either hormone ablation therapy (see chapter 9) or painkillers and other medications if he was at the end of life. "Conservative therapy" is another term that, while not widely used, refers to the avoidance of surgery or radiation. This strategy is also referred to as "expectant management," which implies that something will happen in the future and the task is to "expect" this. Today we talk about "delayed or deferred therapy" or "active surveillance." The premise of delayed/deferred therapy is that of buying quality time for the man at his existing level of functioning and with his existing quality of life. Delaying therapy is usually done using an active surveillance approach. As you will read in upcoming chapters, one of the hallmarks of treatment for prostate cancer is a resultant decrease in quality of life due to the short- and long-term side effects of the various treatments. Delaying treatment, for even two or three years, can have benefits for the man and his partner/spouse. Think of it as buying quality time.

WHAT IS INVOLVED IN ACTIVE SURVEILLANCE?

Much of the information in the following section is going to be quite technical, and you may wonder why you need to know this. The reason is simple: most couples are quite shocked when told that there is no need to treat prostate cancer. How can this be true? Most of us believe that if cancer is found in the body, it must be gotten rid of immediately and completely. So it can be very difficult to understand how and why a health-care provider might suggest to someone you love that he not have any treatment immediately, and perhaps not at all. The doctors should discuss the reasons for this with all patients and their partners, but it is easy to get confused and not hear all the details. So what follows is a presentation of what we know about delaying treatment using an active surveillance strategy.

Dr. Laurence Klotz, a urologist from Toronto, has been a leading expert in active surveillance for many years. According to him, this is a good strategy for men with low-risk disease where active treatment can be provided if and when certain criteria are met.[1] He supports the use of active surveillance in these men for the following reasons:

1. Men with low-risk prostate cancer are easy to identify with some accuracy based on their Gleason score.
2. There is no treatment for low-risk cancer that has minimal side effects and costs.
3. If these men do progress, there is still time to treat, and there are treatments available that are effective.
4. The psychological effects of living with untreated cancer have less effect on quality of life than any of the established treatments offered to the patient.

At the time of writing, there are no clearly established criteria by which physicians monitor patients on active surveillance or even for which men can be offered this strategy. Some physicians base their decision to offer surveillance on the estimated years that the man may live after diagnosis; more than ten years usually means that the patient will be offered active treatment, but less than ten years means that he would be recommended to just watch the cancer. There are obvious pitfalls with this approach; it is not always easy to make this estimate of longevity, and physicians can be wrong in their estimation. There are some protocols that have been used in both clinical practice and research studies, and once we have the results of these trials we may have stricter guidelines for how to do active surveillance. In the meantime, this is what we know:

- Active surveillance can be used in men over the age of sixty-five with low-risk disease (Gleason score $\leq$ 6) or in men with a Gleason score of 7 who are older than seventy-five years.
- The PSA level should be less than 10 ng/ml.
- The clinical stage should be T1c–T2a.
- No more than one-third of the samples from biopsy should contain cancer.
- No sample should contain more than 50 percent cancer.
- The man should have a PSA test every three to six months.
- He should have a digital rectal exam at the same time.
- He should have a second biopsy one year after his first biopsy and every year or two after that.
- If there is a significant change in his PSA at any time, another biopsy needs to be done.
- If there is a significant change in the biopsy results (more positive samples or a higher Gleason score), then treatment should be offered.

Today, almost 70 percent of new prostate cancer patients are diagnosed with low- or intermediate-risk disease (Gleason 6 or 7), and very few of them will die of prostate cancer. Almost two hundred thousand new cases of prostate cancer are diagnosed in the United States each year, and most of them (almost 90 percent) will have active treatment shortly after diagnosis and are then left to endure side effects for many years. It is estimated that up to 60 percent of new prostate cancer patients may not require active treatment.[2] In one review, although 40 percent of men meet the criteria for active surveillance mentioned above, less than 10 percent of men opted for this strategy. Put another way, there has been a 30 to 45 percent increase in the number of men diagnosed with low-risk prostate cancer in the past ten years at the same time as there has been a twofold decrease in the use of active surveillance as a treatment strategy. At the same time, the use of brachytherapy (see chapter 6) and androgen deprivation therapy (see chapter 9) has increased by 300 percent.[3] So while the number of men who could be treated at least initially with a conservative approach of no active treatment has actually increased, fewer men are being offered this approach, and some kinds of treatment have actually increased.

HOW SAFE IS ACTIVE SURVEILLANCE?

Safety is an important factor to consider. Like many spouses/partners, you may find the idea of "doing nothing" to be completely unacceptable. Most of us think that immediate treatment is the only way to go if cancer is diagnosed. That is true for many cancers, but because prostate cancer tends to be slow growing and is often not lethal like many other kinds of cancer, holding off active treatment may be appropriate for certain men. Each cancer is different and individual responses to cancer are different too, not only in how the person with cancer responds to treatment but also how the person with cancer responds to the diagnosis. It's not uncommon for the man to agree to active surveillance and have his family react with shock and horror.

James is sixty-five years old. He was not surprised when he was diagnosed with prostate cancer; his family doctor had been watching his PSA levels for more than five years, and they had been rising steadily. His third biopsy in as many years showed that he had prostate cancer. His initial response was panic, but the urologist told him to think about his treatment options after reading some material he was given and to come back in a month to talk about what he wanted to do.

"My advice to you would be to just watch it for a bit," Dr. Sloan said. "It's very early; it's very small and of low grade. It may never progress any further, and

if we don't do anything, you'll be spared a whole host of side effects. But you don't have to rush into a decision. You have time to think about what you want to do."

This helped him to calm down a bit; if the specialist thought he could wait a month before deciding on a treatment—and maybe he didn't need to have any treatment—then surely there wasn't any need for panic.

His wife did not see it the same way. She cried for what seemed to James to be about a week, and then she marshaled their children together on a Sunday afternoon to "talk their father into doing something immediately." That's how Bobby and Belinda, their thirty-year-old twins, described it to him.

James shook his head; this is how Mona typically dealt with things, bringing in her support team and hoping that they could persuade him. But he'd read all the books and pamphlets that Dr. Sloan had given him—and he didn't like what he read. Peeing his pants? Never having an erection again? Bleeding from his rectum? None of that sounded like something he was interested in, and he just wished that Mona could see it that way. He was in for a long fight.

The outcomes for men on active surveillance are good. In a study of older men (aged sixty-five to eighty years) on active surveillance who were followed for twelve years, only 2.1 percent of the men in the study died of prostate cancer.[4] This is the same as the number of treated men who die of this cancer. In another very large study of over fifty thousand men, more than half the men who deferred treatment remained alive and without treatment 7.7 years later.[5] In a Canadian study, overall survival at eight years after diagnosis was 85 percent; however, not all of the men who were deceased died of prostate cancer.[6] Most of the men died of other causes such as heart attack or stroke. The key in monitoring these men is to enable those with less severe disease to avoid treatment while at the same time being able to identify those who will see their disease progress and offering them effective treatment in a timely manner.

WHY DO MEN STOP ACTIVE SURVEILLANCE?

Perhaps a better way of phrasing this question is, why do some men not go on active surveillance? There are a number of reasons for this. The first is that the man may not be told that this is an option for him. While we would like to think that all physicians practice according to the best available evidence and standards of the day, that is not entirely accurate. Some physicians hold very firm beliefs about prostate cancer, and for them there is no such thing as delaying treatment or monitoring the man with prostate cancer. So they will not even talk about it to their patients, even those for whom it may be the best strategy. We don't have very strong evidence (although the evidence is growing) about this treatment strategy, so some physicians may not want to offer it to their patients until they have overwhelming evidence. As you will see in chapter 7, there is often acceptance of new treatments that also don't have good evidence supporting them—but when there is profit to be gained, evidence may be overlooked. There may be a fear that if the patient's cancer gets worse or if the man dies of his cancer, the doctor may be held responsible, and fear of being sued is a powerful influencing factor. Some have even suggested that men who want to follow an active surveillance path should sign consent just as patients do before surgery.[7]

Recent research suggests that the most influential factor in a man deciding to go on active surveillance is the way it is described to him by the specialist.[8] The rationale for active surveillance must be communicated in a way that the patient understands so that he (and his family) does not feel like "nothing is being done." Education is always important, but perhaps even more so in prostate cancer where there are a multitude of choices every step of the way. This is another area where you as the spouse/partner can be helpful—searching for information and learning about this treatment strategy (and all the others too) is a vital role that you can play.

Another important barrier may be that the man's family (and in particular his spouse/partner) does not support him in his wish to delay treatment or avoid it completely. This is usually because family members don't understand what active surveillance is, and like many people, they believe that all cancer should be treated aggressively. This is done out of love and not out of a wish to see the man suffer from side effects. Most people know very little about cancer (or any other illness) until they or someone they know is diagnosed. You may not be aware of the details of prostate cancer in general, or the specifics of his cancer and the side effects of treatment and their effect on his quality of life. This is another reason why it is so important to go with him to all his medical appointments.

Shortly after he was diagnosed with prostate cancer, Larry's doctor persuaded him to go on a clinical study that was looking at active surveillance compared to immediate surgery in men with low-risk prostate cancer. As a university professor, he was happy to participate in research, and he understood very well what it meant to be randomly assigned to one arm of the study. In his case he was assigned to the active surveillance protocol. This did not make his wife, Leslie, very happy, but he had agreed to be part of the study, and this is where he ended up. After eighteen months on the study, his PSA went from 3 to 5.5, and this worried him. He talked to his urologist about it, and Dr. Bradley explained that according to the study protocol, his rising PSA meant that he was at the threshold of needing another biopsy, which would give them a better idea of what was happening in his prostate. Larry agreed to the repeat biopsy, which showed that he now had four out of twelve samples with cancer. He didn't wait to talk to his wife about this and agreed with Dr. Bradley that his time of active surveillance was over and he wanted to have his prostate removed.

He had the surgery two weeks later. A week after that he was shocked to learn from Dr. Bradley that the pathology report from his surgery showed that the cancer was much more widespread than the biopsy report indicated. One of his lymph nodes was positive for cancer. Had he made a terrible mistake by waiting? Dr. Bradley reassured him that being in the study had not jeopardized him in any way. But his wife was less supportive.

"You stupid, stupid man!" she cried when he came back from his appointment. "You never listen to anybody! I said at the time that you should have surgery, but would you listen? Oh, no! I'm not important; the kids are not important. You're the only one who's important—you and your hotshot research buddies!"

Larry had no answer for her. He knew her outburst was because she was scared and she loved him. But he was scared too, and what he most needed now was her support and understanding. He had never felt so alone in his whole life.

PATIENT AND PARTNER FACTORS IN ACTIVE SURVEILLANCE

For some men, quality of life is more important than longevity; each man will make a decision about whether to have active treatment or not based on his own unique values and principles. Hopefully these same values and principles are shared or at least respected by his spouse/partner and family. Men who pursue active surveillance and who receive ongoing support and education from a health-care provider appear to be happier, with better quality of life, and have less confusion about the process.[9]

For some men, being on active surveillance is anxiety provoking, and they find it difficult to live with the uncertainty of not knowing if the cancer is growing or spreading. Men may also worry that they could miss the opportunity to be treated and then face a situation in which they have limited options. Because this tends to be a slow-growing cancer, any changes should be picked up with the careful monitoring that is the basis of active surveillance.

On the other hand, other treatments are being tested all the time, so waiting may actually increase treatment options for men. But for some men and their partners, not having definitive treatment seems to represent uncertainty, and as discussed in the previous chapter, most of us don't like living with uncertainty. Some men find themselves getting very anxious days before they are due to have blood drawn for a PSA level, and their anxiety remains high until they hear the results of the blood test. Of course, if the news is not good and they need further investigations, their anxiety will remain high. But if the results of the test suggest that the cancer is under control and not growing, their anxiety drops, until the next time.

In one study, 81 percent of men who elected to have treatment while on an active surveillance protocol said they chose to have treatment on the recommendation of their treating physician.[10] When their medical records were reviewed, only 24 percent had evidence of disease progression (rising PSA levels or disease progression on biopsy). This may suggest that the physician took their anxiety levels into consideration and suggested active treatment or that the men preferred to "blame" their physicians for the decision to have active treatment.

Simon knew one thing for sure when the specialist told him he had prostate cancer: he did not want to have surgery. His brother had had the surgery two years ago, and he'd told Simon that since that day, he'd not had an erection. Simon couldn't wrap his head around that. No erections? For two years? Simon had been divorced for almost a year, and just last summer he'd met Jeannie, a wonderful woman who'd changed his life. His ex-wife hadn't really liked sex—at least that's how it appeared—but Jeannie was something else entirely! He felt like an eighteen-year-old, and since they'd been together, he felt like a new man.

So when he went back to see the urologist, he told him straight—no surgery, no radiation. He just wanted to watch the cancer and live his life.

But that was easier said than done. He found that a couple of weeks before he needed to have his PSA measured, he got really anxious. He didn't sleep well, and he was really irritable. Luckily his results were good, and the relief he felt when the doctor told him that his PSA hadn't gone up was enormous. But he didn't know how long he could keep this up—the sleepless nights for two weeks before the test and then another week of worry till his doctor's appointment. Jeannie suggested that he talk to the doctor about this; maybe he had seen this in other patients.

He had, and he also had a suggestion. There was a social worker at the same clinic as the doctor who ran a support group for men on active surveillance, many of whom had the same problem as Simon. The doctor told him there was even a name for it—PSA-itis! Even though he didn't see himself as someone who would go to a support group, Simon thought he would give it a try. Maybe he could learn something from these other guys, and it felt good to know that he was not the only one who acted like this.

Studies are mixed on whether being on active surveillance increases anxiety and distress for men. When men are asked specifically if they are stressed or worried, they may answer that they are. But when anxiety and depression are measured using standardized tests, their levels are low.[11] Men who are pessimists to begin with tend to experience more worry and distress, so perhaps the physician needs to take into account the kind of person the man is before offering active surveillance as a treatment strategy.[12] Younger men were more anxious in another study, and the longer they were on active surveillance, the greater their distress.[13] But overall, the number of men experiencing depression or anxiety was not different from the general population in this study.

In a study of older men on active surveillance, some experienced persistent worry, altered mood, and decreased social activity, and some second-guessed themselves about their decision.[14] Others focused on the positive, stating that their good health was a positive factor, and minimized the threat from cancer. Their belief that they were likely to die of something else shored up their optimism, and some took this as an opportunity to see their lives differently and appreciate the fragility of life.

Men who use active surveillance as a springboard to making changes in their life appear to experience less stress. In a study of the effects of lifestyle changes on stress, men who ate a low-fat, vegan diet and who exercised and took part in stress management strategies were found to experience better quality of life in addition to lowered stress.[15] Making this kind of change is quite dramatic and requires a great deal of support from one's partner/spouse. But this is an area where spouses and partners often want to make a difference; helping men to eat a healthy diet and maintain a healthy lifestyle with exercise is a useful strategy and one that may improve quality of life for the partner too! This is shown in another study of men on active surveillance where spouses played a central role in what the man ate and in his use of dietary supplements. In this study, men explained how their spouses controlled that aspect of their lives and how they shared information about diet with each other as they worked toward the goal of keeping him as healthy as possible while on active surveillance.[16]

So while some men do experience stress while living with active surveillance, other men take this monitoring in their stride and don't get anxious or concerned. As the partner of either of these kinds of men, it's important to find a way to deal with your own feelings of uncertainty or anxiety. Uncertainty can be used for a positive change in life and one's relationship, and some couples choose to use this experience as a life-affirming experience and one that offers an opportunity for growth. If you are the one who usually sees the negative side of things, you may not be able to support him in his decision and may cause him to second-guess his decision.

While his actions obviously affect both of you, ultimately it is his body and his life. Do an internal check to see what it is that is bothering you. Are you fully informed of the pros and cons of his decision? Can getting more information help you to better understand why he has decided to do this? Would it help you to talk to another man's partner to see things from someone else's perspective or to just share your worries? Perhaps you just need some more time to see with your own eyes that he is doing okay.

In my practice, I see many couples whose immediate instinct is to "take it out, and take it out *now!*" They tell me that sex doesn't matter, that not being able to control one's bladder is a minor inconvenience compared with the man being dead. But the choice is not death versus erectile problems or incontinence. The choice is often between life with erectile problems and incontinence and life without these problems, whether temporary or permanent. This desire to do something immediately is most often a reflection of their panic and loss of control in the crisis of learning that the man has cancer. If they take the time to find out more, to live with the cancer for a few weeks or months before making a rush decision, the panic usually subsides and is replaced by hope and an ability to see more than a choice between death and quality of life. Active surveillance offers some couples a continuation of that hope and good quality of life.

WHAT COMES NEXT . . .

In this chapter you have read about one treatment strategy—active surveillance. But not every man has low-risk prostate cancer, and for these other men, active treatment is advised. In the next chapter you will learn about surgery for prostate cancer as well as about the risks of side effects from this treatment. But you will also learn about what can be done to minimize these side effects, or at least cope with them as a couple.

• 5 •

Get It Out!

Opting for Surgery

Surgical removal of the prostate is a common treatment in North America but one that has significant side effects including incontinence and erectile difficulties. Men often choose this treatment because they think that they don't have to worry about anything after the prostate is removed. However, the side effects can have profound effects on how the man sees himself and his masculinity. Providing support and encouragement as he deals with these issues can be a challenge to his partner/spouse.

The goal of surgery as a treatment for prostate cancer is threefold: first, to remove the cancer; second, to protect urinary function; and third, to preserve erectile function. Sounds simple, right? It may sound simple, but in reality it's not that easy. Let's start with a repetition of the anatomy lesson from chapter 1. The prostate lies deep in the pelvis, under the bladder and in front of the rectum. The gland surrounds the urethra, the tube that carries urine from the bladder through the penis to the outside of the body. It is surrounded on the outside by a spiderweb of nerves and blood vessels; these nerves are responsible for erections, an important part of the man's quality of life and image of himself as a man. Removing the prostate is a complex and delicate operation, especially if the surgeon wants to preserve the man's urinary and erectile function. And to complicate matters even further, there are a number of ways to take the prostate out.

WHAT TYPES OF SURGERY CAN BE DONE?

Four kinds of surgery can be done to remove the prostate gland; these surgeries differ in their technical aspects. The first and most commonly used approach is what is called an open *retropubic radical prostatectomy* (RRP). Quite a mouthful! The word "radical" just means that the whole prostate is removed. This is an important point; many people wonder why you can't just remove the cancerous tissue like they do for other kinds of cancer. The answer to this lies in the nature of prostate cancer as you read in chapter 1. Prostate cancer tends to be found all over the gland (not just in one spot), and so to be sure that nothing is left behind, the whole prostate is removed. This surgery is performed through an incision in the abdomen, starting under the belly button and ending about at the penis. It is called "open" because the surgeon gets to the prostate through this opening in the abdomen. The surgeon makes a cut through the urethra above the prostate (at the entry to the bladder) and another cut below the prostate, and then the two ends of the urethra are sewn together, almost like mending a garden hose. This surgery has been performed for over one hundred years, and most urologists have learned to do the surgery this way. There are certain advantages including being able to remove some lymph nodes at the same time to check whether there has been spread outside the prostate gland.

The second kind of surgery is more modern and is called a *radical laparoscopic prostatectomy*; the surgeon removes the prostate using instruments that enter the abdomen through small incisions; this is sometimes called "keyhole surgery" because most of the incisions are less than an inch long. One of the incisions is made bigger to allow for the prostate gland to be taken out of the body. This operation is also called a "minimally invasive" prostatectomy because of the smaller size of the incisions. Is this kind of surgery better than the more traditional open surgery? The answer is not clear cut. One large study of almost ten thousand men showed that the only benefit to laparoscopic surgery was a shorter length of stay in hospital (two days rather than three), less need for blood transfusion, and fewer infections and lung problems. But in the men who had laparoscopic surgery, the rates of bladder leakage (incontinence) and erectile difficulties were much higher; these are the quality-of-life factors that most men say are the hardest to deal with.[1] You'll read more about them later in this chapter.

In the last decade, some urologists have used a robot when doing this surgery, and then the operation is called a *robotic-assisted laparoscopic radical prostatectomy*. The story about the use of robots in surgery is an interesting one, and it's also important, as many men today are opting for robotic surgery. The robot was originally developed for military purposes. It allows the surgeon to be many miles from the patient because a computer-assisted set of instruments is inserted into the abdomen of the patient, and the surgeon controls the instruments like a video game. The advantages of robotic surgery are the following: improved comfort for the surgeon; high magnification, which increases the surgeon's ability to see into the operative field; and a smoothing out of any movement of the instruments caused by the surgeon's hand movements.[2] But has it improved anything for patients?

This new technology has been adopted widely in the United States and has become a major source of both expense and profit to hospitals. Since 2000, when robotic-assisted prostatectomies started being performed, the total number of surgeries done per year has increased significantly. Most of these surgeries are done at hospitals that have a robot (35 percent of all the hospitals in the United States), and these hospitals did 85 percent of all the prostatectomies in the United States.[3] While it is a good thing that most of these surgeries are being done in a few hospitals where surgical expertise is higher, there is also a problem because in order to remain competitive, smaller hospitals are buying these robots. In order for a urologist to become good at using this new technology, he or she needs to do at least 250 operations using the robot.[4] The problem is that most urologists in smaller centers don't do nearly that many in the course of their entire career! The American Board of Urology estimates that the average urologist performs fewer than twelve prostatectomies each year.[5] Hospitals in both large and small centers are buying these robots and then marketing them heavily to patients in order to offset the substantial costs of the equipment. Each robot costs almost $2 million, with yearly maintenance costs per robot of $150,000 as well as substantial costs for disposable instruments for each surgery performed. The costs are then passed on to patients; a conservative estimate suggests that a robotic-assisted prostatectomy adds $2,500 to the cost for the patient.

Robert had it all worked out—he was going to have the latest treatment by the most expensive doctor, and he didn't care that he had to travel almost five hundred miles to get it. This was the kind of guy he was—fast thinking, fast talking, and fast acting. And he got it done: surgery with the robot just two weeks after he received his diagnosis, home two days later, and back to work two weeks after that. But there was a problem, a big problem. While his energy levels were almost back to normal, the rest of his life wasn't. He could just not get control of his bladder. He couldn't believe how much he was leaking! He flew back to see the surgeon three weeks before he was due to see him—he wanted this fixed and he wanted this fixed now!

The surgeon seemed too calm, too polite, too disinterested.

"Now Robert," he said in a soft voice, "you know we told you this was possible. I admit that I have never seen anyone so upset because most men expect this. It'll get better over the next few months, and if it doesn't, well, we can put in an artificial sphincter."

Robert didn't want to hear any more of this. He stormed out of the office, and he thinks his parting words were something to do with calling his lawyer. The flight back home was terrible—not only did he have to pay to get on the earlier flight, but it was bumpy all the way and he felt quite sick when they finally touched down.

His girlfriend Jan had been calling him every two minutes while he was in the air. He didn't feel like talking to anyone but his lawyer. How could he live for a few days with this constant leakage? And the doctor had said it could be weeks or even months before it got better! He found the package of material that the doctor had given him just six weeks before—the paper now looked too glossy, the words too upbeat—and in disgust he threw them into the garbage. He was going to talk to his lawyer in the morning.

But are the results worth the extra money? The short answer is no. There has only been one good study of robotic surgery compared to laparoscopic surgery, but this new technology has been widely adopted despite a lack of evidence that it is better. Robotic surgery (as well as the regular laparoscopic surgery) takes longer than an open surgery, and the side effects (incontinence and erectile difficulties) are no different.[6] What is even more concerning is that almost 20 percent of men who had a robotic surgery regretted their decision, and 16 percent were dissatisfied with the outcome; those who had robotic surgery were three to four times more likely to be dissatisfied than those who had open surgery.[7] This may be because they had higher expectations based on what they were told or promised by the urologist.

When men are presented with this kind of surgery as an option, or when it is the only kind of surgery performed by the physician he has been referred to, it is very important to ask how many of these procedures the surgeon has done. Anything under 250 surgeries means that the patient is part of the surgeon's learning, and you need to think long and hard about that. Do you want your partner to be part of the surgeon's learning curve? If you don't think it matters, then it may be okay for him to go ahead with a surgeon who is not an expert in the technique. But if that makes either of you nervous, a second opinion may be warranted, or you should seek out a surgeon who is very experienced with this technique. This may mean traveling to a larger center for the surgery, and then you have to consider additional travel costs as well as the inconvenience of being away from home and your supports at a stressful time. This is an important consideration for the partner/spouse. Staying in a hotel or with friends or family in a strange city may not be ideal for you. You have to think about getting to and from the hospital, even if the man is only there for two or three days, and it may be exhausting for you to sit at the hospital and then have to negotiate your way back to where you are staying. And to be without the comforts and security of home is also stressful.

The last kind of prostatectomy is called a *perineal prostatectomy*. Here the incision is made not in the abdomen but rather through the perineum, the area between the scrotum and the anus. It is not used widely, mostly because the surgeon can't remove any lymph glands with this procedure and also because it is not possible to do a nerve-sparing procedure.

Now it's time to think about the side effects of surgery, both short and long term, and how they impact quality of life.

WHAT ARE THE SIDE EFFECTS OF SURGERY?

Any surgery poses risks for the patient in the form of infection, blood loss, and blood clots that can travel to the lungs or heart. A number of things are done to prevent this, including the routine use of antibiotics both during and after surgery, improved surgical technique that reduces the amount of blood lost, and the use of pressure stockings during and after surgery. Getting the patient up to walk soon after surgery helps to prevent blood clots, even though he may not enjoy it! Because of where the prostate is situated in the pelvis, there is a risk of damage to the rectum, which lies behind the prostate. Careful surgical technique can minimize the risk of damaging the rectum and other organs close to the surgical site. Patients and their family are often concerned about pain after surgery. Most men report very little pain because of the use of epidural anesthesia in addition to general anesthetic for the surgery, and the use of patient-controlled pain medication in the IV while he is still in the hospital.

LONG-TERM SIDE EFFECTS

Bladder Control

The most significant issues for the patient and partner are those affecting bladder control and erectile functioning. Let's talk about bladder control first. The medical term for loss of control of the bladder is *incontinence*. There is a significant risk of incontinence after radical prostatectomy because the valve or sphincter that keeps the bladder closed is usually damaged when the prostate is removed. It is difficult to give statistics for how many men experience this because it is defined differently in different studies. The most commonly accepted statistic is that about 95 percent of men will have regained most of their bladder control by one year after the surgery. This may mean that he wears one pad a day for protection, but he does not always wet it; but it may not mean the kind of control he had before the surgery. But—and this is a big *but*—there is significant distress related to this lack of control for the twelve months leading up to the first anniversary of the surgery. So even when studies say that 95 percent of men have control of the bladder at one year after surgery, there has been a lot of suffering and frustration in the days, weeks, and months leading up to that one year.

Glen had always prided himself on being the strongest guy at the gym. He'd been working out since his early teens and was really proud of how he looked. This was important in the gay community, and he knew he could still draw some stares, even at the age of fifty-two. But all of this was in jeopardy thanks to the surgery he'd had two months ago. He'd been diagnosed with prostate cancer, and he had it out just as soon as the urologist could fit him in. He just wanted it over and done with. His eyes had glazed over when the nurse was talking to him before he left the hospital—it was just blah, blah, blah to him—but now he was really worried.

The first time he went back to the gym he leaked urine like crazy. He was wearing one of those adult diapers, and he leaked right through one in the first five minutes on the treadmill. He thought he was going to die of shame! He hasn't been back since. He's fine the rest of the time, and he wears a pad just in case, but he can't face going back to the gym. What if he has an accident? What if someone sees the big bulky diaper? Oh no, he just can't go back, and it feels like his life is completely ruined.

Most men will have a catheter in the bladder for seven to fourteen days after the surgery regardless of the type of surgery they have. The catheter is attached to a bag, and this collects the urine from the bladder. The catheter is necessary to allow for the join in the urethra (remember the garden hose from earlier in this chapter?) to heal; if urine flows over that join, healing won't occur. Many men describe the catheter as being the worst part of the whole experience.[8] They find it uncomfortable if not downright painful, and they find that it limits their physical activity. Some men describe spending time dealing with side effects of the catheter, including bladder spasms and irritation and burning pain in the penis. As the major support person for the man, you may find that it takes a lot of your time helping him to solve these issues, and some partners are intimately involved in helping him care for the catheter as well as helping him with daily showering or bathing. The wife of one of my patients told me that she got up during the night to empty the catheter bag while he was asleep as they were afraid that it would leak during the night.

When the catheter is taken out, for the first few days or even weeks, the man has very little control over his bladder. He will leak urine uncontrollably and this can be devastating to him. Many of the men in my practice say that this is the worst part of the whole process. They say that they feel dirty and childlike, and despite being prepared for this by the nurses who teach them what to expect, they are still shocked and upset.

Men are told to wear some kind of protection—adult diapers, special pads for men, or even women's sanitary pads—to protect their clothes, the bedclothes, and hopefully their dignity, but this can be very difficult to accept even though it is usually temporary. Wives of men often laugh and say, "Now you know what I've been going through after having children." I'm not sure either of the two experiences are acceptable to anyone, and women can and should be more active in dealing with their incontinence.

Most men will see improvement in their bladder control over the weeks and months after surgery. Being dry at night is often the first sign that things are getting better. And then they are better able to control leakage during the day too. Some men are left with leakage when they laugh, cough, sneeze, move quickly, exercise, or lift something heavy. Other men learn to use the restroom whenever they can and keep their bladders as empty as possible to prevent accidents. Restricting the type of fluid that he drinks (beer and coffee seem to be the major culprits for leakage) and not drinking after early evening are other strategies used to control incontinence. Many men continue to wear some form of protection for weeks or months longer than they need to, just in case.

Incontinence can be socially restricting; some men refuse to go out anymore because they are so scared that they will leak or that someone will notice that they're wearing a pad or diaper. This can be very difficult for you, and your world may be restricted because your spouse or partner doesn't want to participate in activities that are part of your life together. There is help however—studies have shown that exercising the pelvic floor muscles both before and after prostatectomy can help the man regain control of the bladder (and it can help you too if you experience this). Pelvic floor muscle training is taught by specially trained physiotherapists. Some physiotherapists use biofeedback where a tracing on a screen shows the man when the correct muscles are being contracted properly. These exercises can reduce the duration and severity of incontinence by up to 20 percent.[9] More invasive treatments for incontinence that lasts beyond a year include the injection of bulking agents around the urethra and additional surgery to place an artificial valve below the bladder.

How can you help your partner through this difficult time? The first thing is to understand why this is happening and to be positive that things will improve. He may be embarrassed to buy pads or diapers, and you can help him with that. Sanitary pads with sticky backs and "wings" work well, especially after the first weeks when diapers may be better for heavy leakage, but in order for the pads to work, he has to wear briefs and not boxers. Covering the bed with a plastic or rubber sheet will protect the mattress from any loss of urine at night. And having a sense of humor can get most couples over even the biggest frustrations. Accidents will happen, and your ability to keep things in perspective is invaluable. Urine is sterile; it's not dirty or infectious. And bedding and furniture can be cleaned with soap and water.

Brian and Josie have always been the most affectionate couple in their circle of friends, and there's a good reason for that. Sex has always been really important in their relationship, and after thirty-five years of marriage, it still is. They were confident that things would be okay after his prostate surgery; they knew they could talk any problems over and find a solution. They waited until after his six-week checkup at the urologist to see how things worked. Brian had taken a sample of Viagra from the doctor, and they joked about it in the car going home. Josie made a special dinner for them—rare roast beef to give him energy, she joked—and he took the pill about an hour later, timing it so that he would be good and ready at bedtime.

    It felt like they were just starting out, they were so nervous. It was nothing like it had been before, but he managed to get maybe three-quarters of an erection—and then as he felt his orgasm start, he was shocked to pee the bed. What? Josie was shocked too, but she leapt out of bed and came back with a bath towel. She cleaned him and the bed with her usual efficiency, and she ignored the tears that inched their way down his cheeks. What was this, and how were they going to get around it?

Something that is not often talked about is leakage of urine when a man has an orgasm. There's even a medical term for it—*climacturia*—but it has not been studied extensively. In one study, 45 percent of men who had surgery two years before reported urinary leakage with orgasm. Most said it only happened occasionally, but 21 percent said that it happened most of the time or always. Just over half the men said it didn't bother them at all, but the other 48 percent said it was bothersome. Of interest is that only 21 percent said that it bothered their partner.[10] Strategies used to control this include emptying the bladder before sexual activity, and some men use condoms. Condoms require a firm erection to be used, so this may cause a problem for men who do not have a rigid erection. Not everyone likes to use condoms, but it is one strategy that can help to decrease embarrassment. Another study suggests that men who experience this kind of leakage are more likely to avoid sexual activity, have intercourse less often (once in six months), and are not satisfied with orgasm. These men are also more likely to be depressed and have lower self-esteem than men who do not have this side effect.[11] All of the men in these studies were able to control their bladder during daily activity, and this was the only time that they had leakage.

In my practice I have seen men who have some leakage when they are sexually aroused as well as with orgasm. For the most part this is not upsetting for their partners, who take this in stride and are more concerned that the man is so upset. Having a soft towel on top of the sheets is often all that is needed to keep the sheets dry. It's mostly the embarrassment that has to be dealt with, and once again, a sense of humor can go a long way in keeping this to a minimum. And a healthy dose of sensitivity helps too.

Sexual Changes

The other very important long-term side effect is *erectile difficulties* or *dysfunction*. This used to be called "impotence," but that term has fallen out of favor as it implies that the man is weak or ineffective. Many of my patients tell me that is exactly how they feel when they're unable to have an adequate erection for months or years after the surgery. In this chapter I will use the acronym *ED* for ease of reading.

There is a long history to this side effect. Prior to the 1980s, the nerves that cause an erection were routinely cut during the surgery to remove the prostate, and that was pretty much the end of the man's ability to ever have an erection again. Then two surgeons described a surgery where these nerves were "spared," and the era of nerve-sparing surgery was born. Many men who are preparing to have surgery are convinced (or perhaps just overly hopeful) that this nerve sparing will mean that their erectile functioning will remain as it was before the surgery. The facts are less optimistic.

Even if the nerves are spared, rates of erectile functioning range from 13 percent to 86 percent after surgery.[12] Surgeons who trained before 1982, when nerve-sparing surgery was first described, may not know how to do this procedure. It's a very technical and delicate procedure that requires great surgical skill—and not all surgeons get it right. When you look at drawings of the prostate gland, the nerves are often shown as bright yellow cords—in reality they are tiny, barely visible, and look nothing like a bright yellow cord!

Most of what you read in patient education materials doesn't reflect this wide range of outcomes. These materials often present an overly optimistic perspective and use words such as "most" and "all"—but do we really know what this means? Many of the studies of ED after prostatectomy are biased in one way or another. Some studies only enrolled men who had a good chance of regaining erectile functioning after surgery, such as young men with good erections before surgery. But this does not reflect most of the men who have prostate cancer. These men are usually sixty years of age and older and may already have some problems with erections due to common medical conditions like heart disease or diabetes. They may be using medications to lower their blood pressure that are known to cause ED. These men are not likely to see a return of erections after surgery if they were having problems *before* the surgery. Studies often don't report presurgery function. Others claim that erections occur but don't report whether erections were only possible after using one of the drugs that help men with erections (Viagra, Cialis, Levitra). This can be very confusing, not only to patients and partners, but even to physicians.

Walter came back to see the urologist six weeks after his surgery. His wife Joan was so embarrassed when he asked about having sex again. The doctor looked at his file and said that Walter was "fine" and that he had "spared the nerves" and things should work like usual.

Well, things were not anything like "usual." Nothing happened the first night they tried, and then Walter insisted on trying again the next morning. And on and on it went. He was like a man obsessed—he kept nagging at her and bothering her, and if the truth be told, Joan had never really liked sex all that much and had just gone along to keep the peace.

But Walter was a man on a mission, and he went to see his primary care provider who gave him some pills, and Walter just kept on trying. When things didn't improve with the pills, he went on the Internet and ordered something that arrived in a brown wrapper.

Joan was not going to try something that came off the Internet, no matter what it was. She made an appointment to see Walter's doctor and was almost pleased when he told her that some of Walter's "problems" could be related to his blood pressure medicine.

That was just the news she wanted to hear! She went home with a game plan; she was going tell Walter to stop with the pills and the Internet because all this sex was bad for his heart! She just hoped he would believe her.

There are a lot of "it depends" when talking about nerve-sparing surgery. Success depends on the age of the man, his erectile functioning before the surgery, and whether nerves on both sides of the prostate were spared (bilateral nerve sparing) or just on one side (unilateral nerve sparing). The decision whether to spare the nerves may be made before surgery based on the results of the biopsy; if there are a lot of samples on one side that have cancer, then the nerves on that side will not be spared because that may mean that cancer is left behind in the tissues. A decision may also be made during the surgery when the extent of the disease can be seen with the naked eye. If there appears to be a lot of disease on one side, then most surgeons will destroy the nerves on that side, just in case there are some cancer cells in the tissues outside the prostate gland. Remember that the surgeon's highest priority is to eradicate the cancer—and that's probably yours too.

What about laparoscopic and robot-assisted laparoscopic surgery? Despite the high magnification used in these surgeries, which should make seeing the nerves easier, studies don't show better results for erectile functioning. In one study, the average age of men was fifty-seven years, and after laparoscopic surgery, 85 percent of men who had both nerves "spared" were able to have intercourse, many with the aid of medications such as Viagra, Cialis, or Levitra (more about that later). However, only 27 percent returned to their baseline level of functioning; that is less than a third of men who were able to function as they had before the surgery.[13] Other studies confirm these results. If the nerves on one side only are spared, only 18 to 50 percent of men see recovery of erections.[14]

This is important if depressing information. But perhaps an explanation of why nerve-sparing surgery is not guaranteed to save erections is warranted to help you understand what happens. Even with nerve-sparing surgery, the delicate nerves are pushed and pulled during the surgery. This results in them going into shock, and they stop doing what they usually do—cause erections. The erections that men typically have during their sleep, four or five a night, are very important in maintaining the health of the tissues in the penis. They bring blood and, most importantly, oxygen to the tissues of the penis, keeping them healthy. When these nighttime erections don't happen, changes occur in the tissues that make them less responsive to signals from the nerves later on when more healing has taken place. This lack of oxygen is also responsible for another side effect that is seen in up to 70 percent of men after surgery—shrinkage of the penis.

This is a shocking realization for most men, even though it may sound a little funny. Women often joke that size doesn't matter—but it can and does matter, especially to some men. One of the first things that the man may notice is that he does not have enough penile length to urinate into the toilet. This is easily solved at home where he can sit down, but it is a real problem when using a urinal in a public restroom. My patients tell me that they also dribble on their clothing and shoes and are very embarrassed about this. So if you notice that your partner's penis is shorter, suggest that he sit on the toilet rather than dribbling on the floor! Be aware that the penis shrinks both in length and in girth, and this may alter sensation for the sexual partner.

We know that improvements in erectile functioning are possible for up to twenty-four months, with little improvement after that, although some studies suggest that things will get better up to four years after surgery. Men who are able to have an erection within the first three months after surgery have the best chance of regaining function. If a man can have an erection in the first three months after surgery without medication, then he has a 92 percent chance of being able to have erections at twelve months. If he can only have an erection with medication, then his chances drop to 72 percent. But those are pretty good odds. These figures come from the work of Dr. John Mulhall of New York's Memorial Sloan-Kettering Cancer Center. He suggests that after twenty-four months, any improvement is from the man's increasing confidence that he will be able to have an erection.[15] This raises an important point—the role that the man's brain or psychology plays in recovery.

Miles had surgery almost three years ago, and he has not had a proper erection since. He and his wife Rachel don't talk about it much; she's had a rough time with the menopause, and they started sleeping in separate bedrooms when her hot flashes got really bad.

In the beginning they tried using the pills for erections, but it just felt weird to have to plan things. He had to be very careful about when he took the pill because Rachel often wasn't interested. She grew up in a strict Catholic home and never really liked sex, and she certainly couldn't talk about it. So having to plan things with the pills just didn't work.

She did make an effort for his birthday because it was important to him, and on their anniversary too. The first time he took the pill it worked, but he was in such a hurry that it wasn't really satisfying for him, and Rachel seemed to be glad that it was over so quickly. The next time, he could tell that Rachel was doing it just to get it over with, and his erection lasted just a minute or two and then it was gone. Since then they had pretty much avoided each other at bedtime; she went to bed earlier than he did, in the spare bedroom, and he stayed up late watching the late-night talk shows. They were like college roommates, and sometimes he thought they stayed together just because she didn't believe in divorce. How had things gotten so bad?

Many men are used to having erections on demand, easily, and without much planning. This spontaneity pretty much goes out the window after prostatectomy. Now anything to do with erections has to be carefully planned and timed. And it doesn't always work, so the man gets despondent and gives up. He may also find that his desire for sex decreases a lot—we call this a reactive loss of desire or libido. This loss of desire then amplifies his ED, and a vicious cycle is set up. Not having consistent success getting and maintaining erections also causes him to doubt his ability and have performance anxiety. This is when he starts thinking negative thoughts or questioning his ability—will I even get an erection? Will it be hard enough? Will it last long enough?—and poof, there it went!

Another important factor in this is how rigid or hard the penis gets. Many studies define an erection as rigidity of about 60 percent, but this may not be hard enough for penetration. Yes, he may have an erection, but he may not be satisfied with it (and you may not be either!), and it may not be sufficient for what you want to do with it. After the surgery, men will also not have any ejaculate or emission because the seminal vesicles are removed along with the prostate. This can have a psychological effect on the man; some of my patients tell me that ejaculation is very important to them and that the absence of this fluid means that they are not a "real man."

The issue of masculinity is an important one. While you may not see your partner/spouse as less of a man if he experiences ED, the man may not see it this way. For many men, the ability to have erections, and penetrative intercourse, is an essential part of being a man and of masculine identity. Some men find a way to compensate for this loss of masculine identity when they experience ED; they may rationalize that erections change with age or that it is possible to give their partner pleasure without penetration, but their difficulties with erections remain a profound loss no matter what their partner tells them.[16]

There is a bright side to this: men can still have orgasms, even without an erection. This confuses many men who have always associated an erection with orgasm. Orgasms have nothing to do with the nerves that cause erections; they are a result of sensation going from the penis to the brain. But some men report that after this surgery, their orgasms feel different. They may be weaker or even absent, or they might even be stronger, to the point that they are painful. This may be a result of a very tight pelvic floor, and the same physiotherapists who treat incontinence can help teach the man to relax his pelvic floor.

What Can Be Done to Help with ED? So what can be done to help the man with ED after prostatectomy? An important first step is recognizing that while the nerves heal, it is important to keep the penis well supplied with blood. This can be achieved by using whatever medications produce an erection and trying to have sex or masturbating often. The early use of medications to promote erections may in fact improve long-term erectile functioning. There are three drugs available now—Viagra, Cialis, and Levitra—and it is important to try all three. But one study showed that after prostatectomy, only 14 to 53 percent of men responded to these medications. This is not very encouraging.

Steve and Paul have lived together for seventeen years. Their world was shattered a year ago when Paul's PSA rose suddenly and he was diagnosed with prostate cancer. Steve is a nurse and has many contacts in the medical field that he used to find the best surgeon for his partner. Surgery was recommended, and he started on a penile rehabilitation program the day that the catheter was removed. Paul is a natural optimist, and he believed from the very first day that they found out about the cancer that he was going to be okay in every way. Steve has seen things go wrong with so many of his patients that he was a little more cautious.

But things seemed to go well; Paul's PSA dropped to zero by his first checkup, and he had very few bladder problems. And the first morning that he woke up with an erection was a happy one. Steve finally was able to breathe a sigh of relief, but there was still some doubt in his mind that he couldn't shake. The first time they tried to make love, nothing worked. Steve tried to act as if it was nothing, but he could see that Paul was really upset.

"It's okay, honey," he whispered to Paul. "Maybe we just put too much pressure on you. It's only been eight weeks, and it might be too early."

"But I thought . . . with the morning erections and everything. . . . I thought I was going to be okay." Paul's voice shook a little.

"How about we try again another time? I'm pretty tired anyway . . . and maybe next time we use a full dose of the Viagra."

Penile rehabilitation is increasingly being used to help keep the tissues healthy while the erectile nerves heal. There is not a lot of research to support this, but it gives some hope with minimal effort. Penile rehabilitation usually involves taking a low dose of Viagra every night before bed. I describe this to my patients as "vitamin penis"—they may not see any results, much like we don't feel any different when taking a multivitamin every day. But this low dose appears to be enough to protect the delicate tissues of the penis from being deprived of oxygen while the nerves heal. I also encourage men to try to actively get blood into the penis by stimulating it every day in the shower or by involving their partner/spouse in this activity. Some physicians prescribe penile injections three times a week, which has been shown to improve erections, but this evidence is not strong. Many men don't like the idea of sticking a needle in their penis, but it is one method that really works. More about that later.

Some men are more interested in getting an erection just for the purposes of sexual activity and may not want to take any medication on a nightly basis. One of the most common problems I see is men who do not respond to the oral medications because they are not taking them properly. There has to be physical stimulation of the penis in order to get blood into the penile tissues. Taking the medication and then waiting for an erection does not work! Keep reading to learn more.

Here is some information about the three different medications and how to take them properly. One of the most important factors is communication. While most men do discuss their plans for sexual activity with their partner, some don't and take medication, and then their partner goes out for the evening! We'll talk more about communication later in this book, but it is really central to sexual recovery for the man.

Oral Medications These drugs are called PDE5 inhibitors. They prevent blood from leaving the penis once it has entered the tissues following physical stimulation of the penis. This is important information—without physical stimulation, blood will not enter the penis, and an erection will not happen. This is the least invasive method of treating erectile difficulties and is usually the first treatment suggested. The three medications that are available are very similar but have some unique differences from each other.

- Viagra (sildenafil) usually works in thirty to sixty minutes. If taken after a fatty meal, it may take longer to work. It remains effective for four to six hours.
- Cialis (tadalafil) works within about thirty minutes and remains effective for as long as thirty-six hours. It may be taken with or without food. This medication should only be taken every second day (forty-eight hours after first taking it), as it remains in the bloodstream for an extended period of time.
- Levitra (vardenafil) becomes effective in about twenty-five minutes and remains effective for about four to six hours. It should not be taken after a high-fat meal.

If the man is on certain heart medications (containing nitrates), he should not take these medications as they may cause a drop in blood pressure. Visual changes (flashing lights, blurred vision) may be experienced after taking these medications. These medications will not work if they are taken without genital stimulation to move the blood into the penile tissues. These medications should also be taken on at least six separate occasions before deciding that they don't work. Switching to one of the different brands may result in a better result.

You have already read that only up to 53 percent of men respond to oral medications to help them have erections. If these pills don't work, many men are reluctant to seek other help or perhaps don't know that there are other options. In one study, men waited more than two years to seek help after the pills didn't work for them.[17] Of note in this study is that those couples who saw a sex therapist reported an improvement in their sex life, even if the man wasn't able to have an erection. The other options for achieving erections are more mechanical or invasive.

Penile Self-Injection Therapy   This involves injecting a small amount of medication into the side of the penis that causes a local response in the tissues of the penis and leads to an erection. The man may not experience any feelings of sexual excitement but will still have an erection. It may take some time and a number of attempts to find the correct dose of medication that will work. There is a risk that some scarring will occur where you place the needle, and the man is encouraged to switch the site where the needle is inserted. If scarring does occur, it can cause pain and some curving of the penis. There is also a risk of an erection that does not go down in four hours (this is called priapism). This needs to be treated urgently at the emergency room. Failure to treat this condition may lead to permanent tissue damage. This is a very effective method of getting an erection and will even work in men who did not have nerve-sparing surgery. Men are often horrified at the thought of sticking a needle in their penis, but it works; and sometimes they have to be desperate enough to try and are then very happy with the results. Some men find it easier if their partner injects them—and most partners are willing to do this. I have, however, found that some partners think that this is an extreme measure, but ultimately it is a decision that you should make together and hopefully you can come to agreement! A recent study[18] suggests that men are more likely to use this treatment for ED after surgery if their partner is interested in maintaining their sexual relationship. The partner's motivation in this study was directly related to the presence or absence of their own sexual problems. So if the woman has no interest in sex or is experiencing other sexual problems (such as vaginal dryness after menopause), she is less likely to support and encourage her male partner to use injections to get erections.

Intraurethral Therapy   This method involves inserting a small pellet of medication into the opening of the penis using a special applicator. Once the pellet has been inserted, there needs to be physical stimulation of the penis in order to disperse the medication. After taking this medication, some men experience burning inside the penis or when they pass urine.

Vacuum Therapy This therapy involves the use of a special vacuum device that draws blood into the penis. A tight rubber band is placed at the base of the penis to trap the blood in the tissues. The device can remain in place for thirty minutes and must then be removed to avoid damage to the tissues. Some men find that they have bruising of the penis after using this, and sometimes the penis feels cold to the touch, which some partners find uncomfortable. It takes some dexterity to use this device, although a battery version is available that is easier to use than the hand pump.

Surgical Implant If none of the methods discussed above work, some men may consider having a permanent surgical implant inserted. A surgeon places two cylinders into the penis which are inflated by activating a small pump in the scrotum when the man wishes to have an erection. The insertion is done under general anesthetic and has the usual risks of surgery; however it is a permanent solution. Most men who have this surgery are very happy with the results. It does need to be done by an experienced surgeon, and most implants have to be replaced after about ten years. It's also expensive, but it works!

Finding Help It is universally accepted that men and their partners need additional information about sexual function in the months after surgery. While information is given in copious amounts before surgery, it is not clear how much is retained or understood in the days leading up to surgery. So it is very important for health-care providers to give patients and partners information after treatment when they may be better able to understand and retain the information. This is especially true for information about sexuality.

Studies have shown that men are hopeful that erections will return, and for some, their actions are left at that: hope without help seeking. In a study mentioned earlier in this chapter (see note 16), 35 percent of men who did not respond to oral medication for ED rejected the offer of other options by their physician; they stated that they preferred to wait for things to improve by themselves. The role of the partner in motivating men to try something else or to stick with a certain treatment was important; in 48 percent of the couples in this study, it was the female partner who made the decision to accept help.

While your partner's health-care providers may not offer help for erectile problems spontaneously, they will answer any questions you may have. It's a strange thing, but we know that health-care providers are often reluctant to talk about things related to sexuality even when sexual changes are expected due to treatment. So it's often the patient or his partner who has to raise the topic.

There is help available for couples facing sexual challenges after prostate cancer. There is a specialized field of medicine called sexual medicine, and experts in this area have interest and expertise in treating couples with problems. Some nurses and physician assistants also have an interest in this area—these professionals who often work alongside the urologist may be your best bet for finding help. They can often deal with the issue themselves or refer you to a sexual medicine specialist or sexuality counselor or therapist.

Sexuality counselors and therapists bring a broad and holistic approach to treating couples who are experiencing sexual difficulties. They do not rely solely on medication but instead focus on the couple's unique circumstances and history. Their focus is often on finding different ways for the couple to be sexual together, taking into consideration their past patterns and habits. Many people think that sex therapy involves nudity, but this is a myth. Sex therapy is a solution-focused approach that stresses communication and new behaviors to overcome difficulties.

Problems Passing Urine

Some men (up to 22 percent) develop scar tissue where the two ends of the urethra are sewn together. This is called a bladder neck contracture or stricture and may make it difficult or impossible for the man to urinate. What generally happens is that over time his stream of urine gets weaker and weaker. It's important to report this to the surgeon, as the only thing that will help is to try to dilate the area to allow urine to flow freely or to have laser surgery to get rid of the excess scar tissue.

HOW DOES THIS AFFECT YOU?

You have read in this chapter about the challenges of short- and long-term side effects of surgery, and brief mention has been made about how the partner feels or acts. Cancer can bring a couple closer together, and many couples discover that this is true. After going through the various stages of cancer, from diagnosis through treatment and recovery and into survivorship, many couples find that their bond is even stronger. In a study of couples' agreement on key issues related to prostate cancer, 92 percent of men and women felt that their relationship was better and stronger than before. In this study, most couples (71 percent) said that their sexual relationship was important before treatment, but this dropped to 60 percent after treatment. So couples adapt to the sexual changes brought about by treatment, but 90 percent of these couples felt that the woman's support was critical to helping the man restore sexual function.[19]

Just as information is important to the man with prostate cancer, your needs for information are very important too. A study has shown that older women in particular have greater unmet needs when it comes to information.[20] The topics where unmet needs were highest in this study were what to do for the man when he was discharged from the hospital, how best to provide emotional support to him, how to find help with financial and household problems, and how to approach sexual changes. This is another reminder of how important it is for you to go with him to all his medical appointments, because it is there that the most information will be provided.

WHAT COMES NEXT . . .

This chapter has provided you with a detailed overview of the benefits and risks of surgery to remove the prostate. It's a lot to take in, and you may want to reread sections both before your partner/spouse makes his decision and after he has surgery. There are still other options to consider, and the next chapter describes the pros, cons, and quality-of-life side effects of radiation therapy, another tried and trusted treatment for prostate cancer.

· 6 ·

What about the Noninvasive Route?

Radiation Therapy

*E*xternal beam radiation and brachytherapy are the most common forms of radiation used to treat prostate cancer. Side effects include urinary and bowel problems and to a lesser extent erectile difficulties. This chapter will highlight what is involved with these treatments and how the partner/spouse can support the man as he goes through treatment and recovery.

Radiation is a commonly used treatment for prostate cancer that has been around for many years. It is sometimes reserved for older men or for men who can't have surgery because of the risks of general anesthesia. But there are also some men who don't want to have surgery for any number of reasons and prefer the idea of a noninvasive treatment like radiation therapy.

It is also given to men after surgery to remove the prostate whose PSA continues to rise; when this happens, a recurrence is suspected. All men, regardless of treatment type, will have their PSA levels monitored for many years. The PSA is more accurate after treatment than before as a measure of whether there is any cancer left in the body. The PSA level should be at or very close to zero after surgery, and if it is not or if it rises over time, then further treatment is needed because not all the cancer was eradicated. This is usually done with external beam radiation with or without androgen deprivation therapy. The radiation is not targeted at the prostate itself because it is no longer there, but rather at the area where it used to be, which is called the "prostate bed." This is called "adjuvant radiation therapy."

Radiation therapy is given in different ways: by external beam, brachytherapy (seed implant), and a couple of newer methods (CyberKnife, proton therapy) that will be discussed in chapter 7. The side effects are the same for all kinds of radiation, and they are discussed a little later in this chapter. Radiation therapy works by preventing cancer cells from reproducing. It is more effective with fast-growing cells (cancer cells) than slower-growing cells (normal cells), and in this way the cancer is stopped in its tracks. Let's start by talking about external beam radiation.

EXTERNAL BEAM RADIATION

In this treatment, a linear accelerator (a big machine) turns around the patient, who lies on his back on a narrow table. The linear accelerator sends beams of radiation to the prostate gland, and it moves in a 360-degree circle around the man so that the whole prostate is treated. This treatment is given every day for six to eight weeks, and the treatment itself takes about ten minutes. The man doesn't feel anything while it is happening. Today, most radiation treatments are done using 3D-conformal radiation therapy (3D-CRT). A sophisticated computer program is used to plan where the radiation beams will go, and every effort is made to avoid structures close to the prostate; they try to protect the rectum and the bladder. In this way they minimize damage to these organs and as a result keep side effects to a minimum. A newer form of 3D-conformal radiation therapy is intensity modulated radiation therapy (IMRT). Using even more sophisticated computer programs, different amounts of radiation are given to different areas of the prostate. This allows for maximum targeting of cancer cells while sparing areas of the prostate that do not have cancer, and of course protecting other organs in the area like the bladder and rectum from radiation damage.

Some radiation oncologists place tiny pieces of metal in the prostate before treatment begins to help guide the beams to the prostate. These are called fiducial markers, and when used with IMRT, they enable image-guided radiation therapy (IGRT) to be given. This allows for even more accurate treatment because the markers allow the radiation oncologists to see if the prostate has moved or shrunk as sometimes happens during treatment, and it increases the accuracy of the treatment.

Take notes of these terms and ask your partner's radiation oncologist if this is what he/she does. If the answer is no, ask why not. The reason may be that the cancer center doesn't have the necessary equipment or the radiation oncologist doesn't have experience with these newer treatments. That may be a good reason to get a second opinion at another cancer center.

BRACHYTHERAPY

In this form of radiation therapy, tiny seeds containing radioactive iodine or palladium are inserted into the prostate itself, and over time, the radiation given off by the seeds prevents cancer cells from reproducing. The word "seeds" doesn't quite describe what these sources of radiation look like. They really look like short pieces of pencil lead, about a quarter of an inch long. The seeds are implanted directly into the prostate while the man is under general anesthetic. The seeds are left in the prostate to do their work. Gradually the amount of radiation given off by the seeds diminishes until they are inert or inactive. This means that after about six months the radiation is done, and the treatment is over. Brachytherapy is sometimes given to men in addition to external beam radiation; this is called a "brachy boost."

Brachytherapy is not suitable for all men with prostate cancer. It is usually offered to men with low- or intermediate-risk prostate cancer with a PSA of less than 10 and with moderate-volume disease (half or less of the samples taken). The prostate can't be too big or too small, but if it is large, a short dose of androgen deprivation therapy (see chapter 9) will shrink the prostate enough for the man to be able to have the procedure. It is also not usually advised for a man who has a lot of urinary problems, as the radiation will only make his symptoms worse.

WHAT ARE THE SIDE EFFECTS?

External beam radiation and brachytherapy have similar side effects, but their onset is different. Let's start with EBRT first. Every day that radiation is given, the amount of radiation is added to that of the days before, so we say that the dose is a cumulative one. This also means that any side effects tend to start later in the course of treatment rather than at the beginning. Most men only start to experience side effects a couple of weeks into the treatment. With brachytherapy, the day that the seeds are implanted is the day that the radiation dose is the highest; every day after that the amount of radiation emitted by the seeds goes down. So with brachytherapy, side effects tend to be almost immediate and decline with time.

It is also important to remember that the age and general health of the man may have an influence on side effects from treatment, so it is important to take into consideration what his functioning is like before treatment. An older man who is already experiencing some problems with his erections may be less bothered by any further changes to his erectile function than a younger man who has good erections before treatment. The same can be said for urinary and bowel side effects; if those problems already exist, this may influence how severe the side effects from treatment are and how much the man is bothered by them.

———∞∞∞———

George is an active fifty-five-year-old marathon runner who had surgery for prostate cancer when he was just fifty-three years old. The cancer came back, and last year he had radiation therapy. He handled it well and worked at his job as a city planner throughout. He was disappointed when he found that he was really tired for the last two weeks of his treatment. He had never experienced this kind of fatigue before—he could barely stay awake after dinner at night, and he had to drag himself out of bed every morning. Running was out of the question, and he was frustrated because he wanted to run in the half marathon to raise funds for the American Cancer Society that was held every summer in his hometown. He hoped that the tiredness was going to be a temporary thing, and his radiation oncologist was noncommittal when he asked how long it would last. To his surprise, it did not end for months. Three months after his treatment was over, he asked again when he would feel more energized. And again he was met with silence and a shrug of the radiation oncologist's shoulders. The other guys that he ran with seemed equally surprised; he'd gone back to running exactly six weeks after his surgery, so why was this taking so long?

Fatigue

About 60 percent of those treated with external beam radiation experience fatigue, and this increases until it reaches its peak as treatment ends.[1] The fatigue does not end with the end of treatment, though. In fact, a very small minority of men (4 percent) reported ongoing fatigue five years after their treatment was over.

What does this fatigue feel like? Some men have described it to me as something that comes from deep inside and that is a unlike anything they have experienced before. It is often relieved by a nap or rest, and usually it doesn't affect his ability to bathe, get dressed, or take care of himself. It may, however, mean that he is too tired to do household chores—and this may cause some friction if those chores then fall on you. He may still have the energy to be active socially, and you may question why he can see his friends for coffee but is too tired to cut the grass! Remember that everyone is different, and there are other factors that influence his fatigue level, including his age, his general health, and any other cancer treatments he may be receiving. In a recent study of cancer patients, men with prostate cancer were the least likely to experience changes to their daily life while receiving radiation compared to people with other kinds of cancer.[2] For men who are on androgen deprivation therapy (see chapter 9) in addition to receiving radiation therapy, the fatigue may be worse or may continue long after the radiation treatment is over.[3]

With brachytherapy, there is less evidence that fatigue is a problem. Many men choose this procedure as a treatment because of the limited time of the treatment (as compared to EBRT), and many go right back to their usual routine within days of having the seeds inserted. Some of my patients report that their physical fatigue is minimal if present at all, but they do have some emotional fatigue once the treatment is over. This is probably related to anxiety about both the cancer and treatment and the relief that treatment is over.

What can be done to reduce this fatigue? As mentioned previously, a nap can help, especially if he takes one just after his treatment. It may also help for him to try to schedule his radiation treatment at a time of day that works best for him in terms of being able to go home and rest. Not all men experience this fatigue or have it so bad that they need a rest. Some of my patients schedule their treatment during their lunch hour and go back to work after they are done.

Exercise can help too, even though this sounds counterintuitive. A small study showed that resistance exercise (weights) as well as aerobic exercise (treadmill or elliptical trainer) helped to minimize fatigue in men receiving radiation therapy. Of interest is that in this study, resistance exercise had the added benefit of improving strength, lowering body fat, and improving quality of life.[4] Another study provides additional proof of the benefit of exercise: prostate cancer patients receiving radiation therapy who participated in a home-based program of resistance and aerobic exercise showed improvements in quality of life and lower fatigue that extended to three months after treatment ended.[5]

This is important information because you can play an active role in helping your partner/spouse get regular exercise—and you benefit too! Exercise has been shown to improve energy levels, and it has a positive effect on mood too. Going for a walk or bike ride together can benefit not just your health but your relationship too—if you turn off your cell phones, you have time together without interruptions and you can talk and support each other. You can also help him to plan his radiation therapy sessions based on when he has the most energy, when he is more likely to be able to rest or nap, or when he needs to conserve his energy for a specific task or event. Most cancer centers encourage patients to be flexible with their daily radiation schedule, and a partner with a day planner or calendar with important events can really help when planning future treatments.

For men who are anxious about radiation therapy, complementary therapies such as relaxation response therapy and Reiki have been shown to lower anxiety levels and increase emotional well-being.[6] This was a small study, but many patients and their partners are interested in complementary therapies.

Urinary Side Effects

Some men decline surgery because they don't want to experience the incontinence that usually follows surgery, as discussed in detail in chapter 5. Radiation therapy can also cause problems with urination, but the two therapies do tend to be different. Men who have radiation therapy may experience urgency and frequency of urination; that is, they may feel the need to empty their bladder more intensely (urgency) and frequently than they did before. They may also experience some pain or burning when they empty their bladder (this is called dysuria). These symptoms tend to occur later in men having EBRT but soon after the insertion of the seeds for men who have brachytherapy. Long-term side effects (these may happen years after treatment is over) may include incontinence (leakage of urine) due to radiation damage to the sphincter that keeps the bladder closed or even some blood in the urine caused by damage to the bladder itself.

In a study of 3D-conformal radiation, 13 percent of patients reported minimal leakage (not enough to use a pad), 90 percent reported needing to pass urine during the night (something that is quite common in men as they age), 30 percent reported the need to pass urine more frequently, and 6 percent reported some pain on urination.[7] Of interest is the finding that despite this percentage of men needing to urinate at night, most of them were not bothered by this. The researchers did not ask the opinion of the spouses of these men who were likely disturbed by their nighttime need to urinate! A newer study of men who had 3D-conformal radiation suggests that effects on the urinary system are minimal, and improvement is seen within two months of the end of treatment and up to one year after treatment is completed.[8]

Stuart had brachytherapy two months ago, and he is finally able to sleep through the night. This is a monumental event because for the last two months, he has been getting up every two hours to urinate. And no one is happier than his partner, Mike. At one point immediately after Stuart had the procedure, Mike had to sleep in the guest bedroom. Stuart was getting up (and waking Mike) every two hours, and Mike was exhausted. He could barely manage to stay awake at work—and as a high school teacher he needed to be awake! Stuart had tried to limit what he drank after 6 p.m., and he even tried a sleeping pill for about a week, but nothing seemed to work. He just had this urge to go every couple of hours—and even then he just produced a tiny amount. His mother suggested that he keep a bottle next to the bed, but Mike drew the line at that. So Mike slept in the guest bedroom, something that he hated to do, and Stuart wore a path in the carpet between his side of the bed and the bathroom. But it was better at last—much better—and Mike moved back to their bed.

———⊂∞⊃———

With brachytherapy, the worst side effects are experienced in the days and weeks following the implant of the seeds, with the greatest bother experienced one month after the procedure and a return to preprocedure functioning by two years.[9]

So what can be done to help with this bothersome side effect? The important point to remember here is that things get better with time; most men return to their baseline level of functioning by two years at the most.[10] There are medications that can help if the man is experiencing an urgent need to urinate—but he has to speak up when he sees his radiation oncologist. This can be a bit of a challenge; I have noticed that men are often reluctant to "complain," and so they don't say anything to the doctor. And that often leaves a frustrated partner or spouse who bears the brunt of his discomfort the rest of the time. This is yet another reason for you to go with him to all his appointments—and to go into the examination room and not just sit in the waiting room. He may not want to complain—but you can explain how side effects are impacting his quality of life, and yours by association!

If the frequent need to urinate is causing problems, there are a few simple actions that can help. Alcohol, caffeine, and spicy foods can cause bladder irritation, which in turn increases the feeling that the bladder needs to be emptied. So restricting these items and seeing if things improve can help. In addition, many men find that if they restrict fluids after late afternoon, they don't need to urinate as frequently during the night so that both of you can get more sleep.

Seeing a pelvic floor physiotherapist can be helpful too. The muscles of the pelvic floor play a vital role in supporting the bladder, and making sure that these muscles are well toned and not too tight or too loose can help with urinary function. It is important to seek help from a physiotherapist who is an expert in working with the pelvic floor; not every physiotherapist has the additional training to do this work effectively.

Another important long-term side effect of radiation therapy is its effects on the bowels and rectum. Let's talk about that now.

Bowel Function

Shirley was one angry woman. She had a short temper at the best of times, but this was enough to push her over the edge. She'd taken care of her husband Tom for the eight weeks of his radiation treatments. He'd been fine most of the time, more tired than usual perhaps, but he hadn't complained much. He didn't want to go out much, and she didn't like this, but after two weeks of nagging him to get out of the apartment, she just started going out herself.

What set her off this morning was the state of Tom's underwear that she found hidden in the back of the closet. There must have been at least eight pairs there, all scrunched in a ball—and they were all soiled. She didn't know what to think or do. Why had he hidden them? Why were they dirty? What was going on? She put them in a pail with half a bottle of bleach and sat on the balcony as she tried to think of a way to broach the topic with him.

But it was Tom who started talking; he'd seen the pail with the soaking underwear in the bathroom, and he was ready to fess up. He could barely look at her when he told her that for the past couple of weeks he'd been unable to control his bowels, and that was why he didn't want to go out—in case something happened when he was out of the house. And he'd hidden his underwear because he was ashamed to tell her. But he hadn't found a moment to deal with them—and he didn't really know how—and now she'd caught him and he felt awful. Her anger melted away as he spoke, and she reached out and took his hand. At least she knew now, and she would help him; of course she would.

Up to 10 percent of men will experience some bowel side effects during and after radiation therapy. It is believed that this side effect is in part dependent on the skill and expertise of the radiation oncologist.[11] Remember that the prostate and rectum are very close together, so it's possible for the rectum to be exposed to fairly high levels of radiation. Some men report some involuntary loss of feces while on radiation therapy; this is usually intermittent, but it does impact quality of life.[12]

This damage to the rectum is called radiation proctitis (inflammation of the rectum), and the symptoms experienced include diarrhea, rectal pain, frequent urges to pass feces, and at times rectal bleeding. These symptoms usually occur gradually and are difficult to live with. If the man already has a chronic condition such as diabetes, the likelihood of having these rectal problems is increased, and healing can take a very long time. Researchers have also found that men who have significant side effects during treatment are more likely to have long-term difficulties.[13]

Radiation proctitis is more likely to happen after external beam radiation than brachytherapy; the newer techniques such as IMRT are said to reduce the number of men who experience this bothersome side effect. If your partner/spouse experiences any of these symptoms, it is very important that he report them because rectal bleeding can also be a sign of colorectal cancer, and one shouldn't assume that the bleeding is only related to the treatment and not to something else. It is not uncommon for men to be on blood thinners or daily aspirin, and these may increase the risk of rectal bleeding during and after radiation therapy,[14] but once again, don't assume that this is the cause and encourage your partner to get checked out.

What can be done about these side effects? As with urinary side effects, it's important for your partner/spouse to report these so that treatment can be given to control the side effects as soon as possible. Changes in diet may be necessary to help with diarrhea and the urgent need to empty the bowels. A low-residue diet will reduce the amount and frequency of bowel movements. Foods to avoid on this diet include whole-grain products, nuts and seeds, vegetables and fruits with their skins on, popcorn, and other foods that are rough or unprocessed. Foods that are allowed on a low-residue diet include white bread, well-cooked vegetables without skins, dairy products such as yogurt and milk, soft eggs, and clear broths.

Sexual Function

Many men, and their partners, are concerned about the effects of any treatment on sexual functioning, and this includes all types of radiation therapy. You've read the statistics on sexual difficulties after surgery, and you will now read about the effects of radiation. Because external beam radiation therapy is often used to treat prostate cancer in older men who cannot have surgery, it can be difficult to interpret the results of many studies on this topic. Many older men already have some degree of difficulty with erections, and so any treatment to the prostate has the potential to make this worse—and it certainly won't make things better! The other factor that causes difficulty with these studies is that radiation therapy is often given with androgen deprivation therapy (ADT or hormone therapy). As you will read in chapter 9, ADT has a profound effect on all aspects of sexual function including sexual desire and erections.

Pete decided to have brachytherapy because he'd read that this was his best option if he wanted to have any kind of sex life. His wife Laura was not 100 percent with him on this—she wanted him alive at any cost. But they were only in their early sixties, and they'd had a great sex life up till then. She knew it was very important to him—and yes, it was important to her too.

He had the procedure, and she was thrilled at how quickly he recovered. Within two days, he was back to his usual energetic self. He wanted to "give it a go" on the third day after the implant of the seeds, but she was not ready. She read all the material that the nurse had given her, and it did say that he could resume sexual activity when he felt ready, but what about the partner? What if she didn't feel ready? They waited a week—a very long week, said Pete—and both of them were a little shocked when his semen was a red-brown color. Laura read the material from the nurse again, and there it was in black and white: the semen may appear discolored for weeks after the implant. She was relieved to read that and to know that nothing was wrong with him, but she was still a little shaken. Pete, however, seemed not to care—she realized that he had been very worried about whether he could "do it," and watching him sleep with a smile on his face made her smile too. He looked so happy, and that was important, very important. But she was going to keep the reading material from the nurse close at hand for a few weeks longer, just in case.

Unlike after surgery, when erections are immediately affected, changes to erectile function in men undergoing radiation therapy tend to occur over one to two years after treatment.[15] Men who have EBRT tend to fare worse than men who have brachytherapy; rates of erectile problems after EBRT are from 6 to 84 percent but much less for brachytherapy (0 to 51 percent).[16] In another study of brachytherapy, while 77 percent were able to have erections sufficient for penetration before treatment started, this percentage had dropped to 50 percent by the end of the five-year follow-up period.[17] 3D-conformal radiation therapy falls somewhere in the middle, with 7 to 59 percent of men reporting erectile problems after this form of radiation therapy.[18]

Radiation also decreases the amount of semen that is expelled with ejaculation, and although most men are not bothered by this, they will notice the change. The semen may appear thicker and over time may disappear completely, leading to what is called "dry ejaculation." After brachytherapy, the semen may appear red or even brown for an extended period. This is because of old blood resulting from the trauma to the tissues of the prostate caused by the needles that were inserted to put the seeds in place. It is similar to the bleeding that occurs after a prostate biopsy. For the first couple of ejaculations, men are advised to use a condom just in case (and this is very rare) a seed comes out with the ejaculate.

Many men think that the changes in their erections are due to age, and because these changes happen over time, they don't link their occurrence with the treatment they had. This may also be due to a lack of discussion about sexual side effects, something that is not uncommon in encounters with medical specialists. A recent study looking at these discussions with patients by both urologists and radiation oncologists found that this topic was not raised in 50 percent of the consultations observed, and the patient or partner hardly ever brought up the topic or asked questions.[19] This may be due to the particular attitudes of the physicians involved—that the patient is too old to be sexually interested or active is a common observation—or the physician may be too embarrassed to talk about it or may feel that it is not part of his/her responsibility.

So what can be done about these changes? On a purely physical level, men who experience erectile difficulties after radiation therapy respond well to medications such as Viagra. In one study, 55 percent of men who took this medication had erections sufficient for successful intercourse more than three years after treatment (compared to just 18 percent of men who took a sugar pill). Two years later, 24 percent of the original men were still using it.[20] It has also been suggested that taking these medications early after treatment (within in the first year) may be of benefit in protecting erectile functioning at pretreatment levels.[21] If the medications don't work, or if the man doesn't like taking them, any of the other erectile aids (the pump or injections) may work.

It is always important to view the man as a whole person and not just as a penis. This may sound funny, but there is much more to a man's sexuality than how his penis functions. When thinking of the man as a whole person, it also means considering his relationship with his partner. I have many patients who desperately seek help for their erectile problems while this is of little concern to their spouse/partner. Sometimes the partner/spouse goes along with the man's wishes, but other times, the partner/spouse is more vocal and will state his/her opinion about using erectile aids. There are many different ways to be sexual as an individual and as a partner, and the focus on the penis as the central aspect of sexuality is perhaps a limited one.

Other Side Effects

Any of the forms of external beam radiation may cause skin damage over the area where the beams pass through the body. This is in part dependent on the man's skin tone, with fair men (especially those with freckles) experiencing the worst skin damage and black men the least. The radiation therapist will give advice on how best to care for the skin over the area, and it is wise to follow his or her advice to the letter. Most men will lose body hair in that area too—but not on the head!

Partner Issues

You have just read about the views of a man's partner when it comes to sexual functioning, but what about other issues related to radiation therapy? One of the most frequent concerns I hear from both my patients and their partners is about radiation exposure of the partner. Are you or anyone else in your family going to be exposed to radiation because your spouse/partner is having radiation therapy? If he is having external beam radiation, including 3D-CRT or IMRT, then the answer is no. The radiation that he receives every day is not given off from his body. Even if he has brachytherapy and the radiation source is inside him, the risks to you and your family are so low as to not be a concern.

Let me explain this: every day we are exposed to radiation in the environment, even if we don't know it. Every year the average US citizen is exposed to 3.60 mSv (this is the measure of radiation), and depending where you live, that dose may be greater. If your partner/spouse has brachytherapy, you may be exposed to 0.10 mSv. Because you are not with him every minute of the day, and when you are, you are separated physically for most of the time, your additional risk from his brachytherapy treatment is no worse than from everyday events that we don't regard as important or even as a source of radiation. Sleeping in the same bed is allowed, although it is advisable not to sleep in the spoon position for any length of time. The same applies to other people in the household as well as pets and friends; casual contact is fine and does not place anyone at additional risk. We are more cautious with pregnant women and small children, who may be more sensitive to radiation; we advise men to avoid prolonged direct contact, that is, close contact (e.g., holding in the lap), for many hours on multiple occasions.[22]

Nate and his wife June are pleased that he finally has a date for brachytherapy after almost three months of trying to make a decision. They tell their daughter Kim, who at twenty-nine is expecting their first grandchild. They didn't expect her reaction.

"What? You can't be serious! Why don't you just have it out? If you have those seeds, I'm not going to be able to see you for the rest of my pregnancy—and you're not going to be able to hold the baby!"

Nate and June looked at her in shock. What was she talking about? Through her tears she told them that she'd been doing some reading on the Internet, and the things she'd read about brachytherapy led her to understand that he couldn't have close contact with a pregnant woman (her) or small children (her baby, due in five months).

"That's not exactly accurate," began June. "The doctors and the nurses say that you shouldn't sit on Dad's lap when you're pregnant, and seeing how big you've grown, I'd worry about Dad's knees."

Her attempt at a joke fell flat, so Nate picked up the conversation.

"Honey, I thought of that. And Mom's right—you can't sit on my lap for an extended period of time, but you don't do that now! And by the time the baby is born my treatment will be long over—and there's nothing that says I can't hold a baby . . . just not for extended periods of time for a month or so afterward. It'll be fine, honey—please believe me."

Kim trusted her Dad, she always had, and she smiled briefly as she wiped her nose with the back of her hand. She loved her Dad so much, and she wanted the best for him. She would listen to him this time and pray that it would be okay.

The issue of radiation exposure is one that causes great concern. In a study of the wives of men undergoing brachytherapy, women reported that they didn't know how to touch their husbands after the procedure.[23] This is likely a reflection of their confusion about what is safe and what is going to endanger them; they have either not been told clearly enough what is safe to do (all daily contact including sleeping in the same bed), or they are overly fearful for their own safety.

Fear of being close to one's partner does not apply to everyone: in a study of almost five hundred men who had brachytherapy, three of the men had made their partners pregnant. The women were significantly younger than the men, and none of the couples had been counseled about contraception. Even though the amount of their semen was decreased, testing showed sperm in the semen that were viable and that obviously resulted in the pregnancy of their partners.[24]

WHAT COMES NEXT . . .

Many men and their partners are very satisfied with the outcomes of radiation therapy. The treatment is non- or minimally invasive, with limited down time for the man. And it is widely agreed that this treatment is just as effective in terms of curing cancer as the more invasive surgery. The next chapter will describe some of the newer kinds of treatment for prostate cancer, some of which are gaining in popularity even though there are no long-term studies to judge their effectiveness.

· 7 ·

Shall We Try This?

New and Experimental Treatments

*E*very week it seems that another groundbreaking treatment for prostate cancer is discussed in the media. Proton therapy, CyberKnife, light therapy, high-intensity focused ultrasound, and cryotherapy—what are these treatments and can they help with the kind of prostate cancer that your partner/spouse has been diagnosed with? How do you separate the myths and the promises from the realities? This chapter will discuss experimental treatments and how to evaluate their worth. You will also read about the most current evidence on the role of diet and exercise in maintaining health for prostate cancer survivors.

Prostate cancer is big business for hospitals and cancer care providers, including surgeons (urologists), radiation oncologists, and medical oncologists. Because the established treatments (surgery and radiation) are equally effective in treating prostate cancer, competition for patients is a significant factor for the bottom line. And of course you have to take into consideration some newer treatments that may be safe but whose effectiveness may be questioned. In this chapter, you will read about a number of treatments that have not yet proved to be more effective than the traditional treatments (surgery, radiation therapy). But there is a lot of hype about these treatments and many men who will testify that X or Y worked well for them, so why should other men not benefit? This is going to be a fairly technical chapter, so take a deep breath and start reading.

CRYOTHERAPY

Cryotherapy (or cryosurgery as it is sometimes called) is not a new treatment, but it is one that is not widely used for a variety of reasons, including side effects and the fact that not many care providers have been trained to use this treatment. Cryotherapy kills cancer cells by freezing them, resulting in cell death when ice crystals form in the cells themselves. Thin needles are inserted into the prostate, and an ice ball forms at the end of the needles when special gases are pushed into the needles. The treatment is done under general anesthetic, and men have a catheter in the bladder for two to three weeks after the procedure. Many patients regard this as a minimally invasive treatment even though general anesthetic is required. It is most often used to treat men who have had radiation therapy and experience a return of the cancer; it is often referred to as a salvage procedure. Some men may opt for this as a primary treatment, but they need to be aware of the effects on erections. For this reason it is mostly offered to men who already have erectile problems and are prepared to accept this permanent side effect.

Rudy came back from his appointment with the oncologist with a satisfied look on his face. He'd been impressed by the young doctor he'd seen, and he told his wife Joan that he was going to have some kind of "freezing" to treat his cancer. Joan was a little confused because the last time they had talked about it with their son James, who was finishing his residency in neurology, Rudy had seemed ready to go ahead with surgery.

"Don't you think you should talk to James about this? He thinks you're having surgery, and I want to know why the change of plan."

"Yeah, maybe I should tell him," Rudy replied.

Joan could hear her son's surprise when his father told him on the phone about the change in plan.

"What? Why? Did he talk to you about the side effects, Dad?"

Rudy admitted that he'd been told very little, mostly about how this could be done quickly—the next week in fact—and he hadn't asked any questions at all.

"I've been doing some reading, Dad, and, well, this cryotherapy will change your life—and not in a good way. You need to do some reading and thinking, and please talk to Mom before you do anything!"

Joan watched as Rudy replaced the phone on its base. He looked a lot less satisfied now, and she went to put the kettle on before they started to talk.

A major drawback to this treatment is that when the prostate is frozen, the nerves responsible for erections are also affected, and up to 90 percent of men will not be able to have erections after the procedure. Some functioning may return; in a small study of seventy-five men, 13 percent recovered erectile function at three years after they had cryotherapy, and a further 34 percent were able to have erections with the help of medications such as Viagra.[1] A more recent study of just fifty-three men showed small and slow improvements in erectile function, with 39 percent able to have erections two years after the procedure.[2] A nerve-sparing approach to this procedure has been suggested with good results in a very small sample of just nine patients. The question that is always raised with nerve sparing is does it also spare cancer as some tissue is not frozen to protect the erectile nerves? Experts are in agreement that this approach needs further study.[3] Incontinence may occur in up to 20 percent of men, but with greater expertise of the physician, this is usually lower, with just 4 percent of men in one study reporting this side effect six months after the procedure.[4]

Many spouses/partners are less interested in sexual side effects than they are in how well the procedure works against the cancer. In a review of studies of cryotherapy, survival statistics indicate that this is an effective treatment, with 92 percent of men surviving to the five-year mark.[5] So this procedure may be right for your partner, or either one of you (or both) may not want to experience the sexual changes that will occur for the man.

If you and your partner think that this is an attractive option for him, ask about it. The urologist he is seeing may not know all that much about it (it is often performed by radiation oncologists even though it is not a treatment involving radiation), but you have every right to seek alternative treatments.

HIGH-INTENSITY FOCUSED ULTRASOUND (HIFU)

HIFU uses powerful ultrasound waves focused on the prostate gland that destroy the tissue. This technology has been around since the 1990s and has been used mostly in Canada, Europe, and Asia. It has never been approved for use in the United States; however, there are a number of centers that are using this technology as part of a clinical trial. One trial compares HIFU to cryotherapy and another to brachytherapy.[6] Because it has never been approved by the FDA, many US men travel to Canada to have this treatment at a cost of about $25,000. Like many of the other new or experimental treatments, advertising by the companies that make the equipment often drives men to want to have what they are offering. And often the claims that are made—"noninvasive treatment that preserves quality of life"—have not been proven. But they sound wonderful, and most of us would like a quick fix with minimal side effects for whatever ails us.

In recent years there have been a number of reviews of all the studies that have been done on HIFU.[7] And each of them says the same thing: the studies of this treatment are limited in number of participants, what they are measuring in terms of effectiveness is not always clear, and the studies have reported on outcomes for a maximum of six years. This does not compare to the many years of outcomes we have for the traditional treatments, and so conclusions about HIFU being as good as surgery or radiation cannot be made.

There was nothing that Carol was able to do to change her husband's mind; Bruce was like that once he decided on something. She was a nurse and had done a lot of research when Bruce was diagnosed at age forty-eight with prostate cancer. Then he found this clinic in Toronto that was doing HIFU, and he decided that this was it. He made plans to go there a week later; Carol couldn't get off work, so he went alone. He came back with a glossy binder full of glowing talk about the treatment. But Carol wanted to know why it was not FDA approved; she felt that something was wrong, but she couldn't quite place where this feeling was coming from.

She went with him to Toronto for the treatment two weeks later. She was nervous the whole time while she waited for him to wake after the anesthetic, and she was really surprised when the nurse in the recovery room started explaining to her how to take care of the catheter. She knew how to do that—but why had Bruce not told her that he was going to have one in the first place? She knew that she had to take it easy with him, but she was angry that he had gone ahead with something that neither of them seemed to know much about.

We know that HIFU is safe, but what about the side effects that impact quality of life? This treatment seems to have better outcomes in terms of incontinence than surgery, but it has higher rates of stricture formation; up to 58 percent of men experience the inability to pass urine over time[8] and need to have the urethra stretched to allow urine to flow. Erectile problems are seen in up to 77 percent of men after HIFU, about the same as with surgery and worse than with brachytherapy.

So why is the interest in HIFU so great that it would prompt men to travel to Canada to have this treatment? In part it may be because it is not available in the United States and so appears to be special in some way. It is a day procedure that takes up to four hours with a general anesthetic, but it requires no hospitalization; the man will have a catheter in place for up to a week. Five-year outcomes suggest that 55 to 95 percent of men are disease free, which suggests that this might be a good treatment for elderly men with a limited life span.[9]

Some people like the idea of being part of something new like an experimental treatment, while others want something that has been tested when treating cancer. So if your partner wants to have HIFU and you think he's taking a chance with his health, what do you do? The ads for this treatment online are very enticing. There are often testimonials from men who have had it who are very happy with their outcomes. But do you think that they would put negative testimonials on the website? Of course not! Would it help to talk to someone who has had the treatment? Maybe, but how do you find these men and their partners to talk to them? Most health-care providers (urologists and radiation oncologists) would not support the use of HIFU because there is not enough long-term evidence to show that it is effective or better than surgery or radiation. Many of the partners of men with prostate cancer that I see in my clinical practice say that it is the man's choice, and they are there to support him in his decision. You read about this in chapter 3, and you may feel the same way. Ultimately it is his body and his choice, but the fallout from his choice will affect you too. This is a difficult position for you to be in. You will read about participation in clinical trials in chapter 10, and perhaps the information in that chapter will help you both to understand the pros and cons when considering experimental treatments.

PROTON BEAM THERAPY

Proton beam therapy is a different form of radiation therapy. It uses protons, which are tiny subatomic particles, to target the organ that has cancer in it. This kind of treatment has been used for years in patients with very rare cancers of the nervous system, but it has more recently gained popularity as a treatment for prostate cancer. The difference between traditional radiation therapy and proton beam therapy is a technical one; radiation therapy tends to spread in the body (much like a beam of light from a flashlight), while the proton beam is more focused on the target organ. So, theoretically, damage to other tissues is much less likely with proton beam therapy.

But this difference in side effects is a theoretical one, and the topic of proton beam versus traditional radiation therapy is controversial and a source of great debate (and argument) among medical specialists. There is virtually no published data from clinical trials that suggest that proton therapy is better than radiation therapy, in particular intensity modulated radiation therapy (IMRT).[10] Most of the studies of this treatment do not compare the outcomes on the patient with traditional radiation therapy, so the benefit to the patient of this therapy is unclear.

Lance and Peter had been fighting day and night since he decided to have proton therapy. Peter had never heard such nonsense in his life, and he was so mad at his partner of thirty-five years that he was barely talking to him. Proton therapy? What the heck was that? He knew that Lance had probably heard about it at the support group he went to. Peter thought it was strange that he was going to a support group that didn't allow partners in the first place—and Lance had always been the first one to mock any of their friends who went to counseling.

And when he saw the material from the hospital that did the proton therapy, he nearly swallowed his tongue—it was going to cost almost $40,000! They didn't have that much money between them and their families. They had just managed to pay off the mortgage on their condo, so how on earth did Lance think he was going to find $40,000 lying around? The whole thing was just incredible to him, but Lance didn't want to talk about it. This was what he wanted, and this was what he was going to do.

So why are we talking about a treatment that is not better than any of the other treatments? Word of mouth is the simple answer. Men are talking about this to each other and encouraging others to have it. There are only five centers in the United States where this treatment is available (with three more under construction and ten more in the planning stages), and perhaps this exclusivity makes it attractive. And of course some men like the idea of being one of the first to have a treatment; this also translates into being a guinea pig, perhaps! Proton beam therapy is very expensive (about double the cost of traditional radiation therapy),[11] and this too may make it more attractive to some men who think that the more expensive something is, the better it is. It costs between $100 million and $150 million to set up a proton beam therapy program,[12] and these costs must be recouped in some way; advertising the therapy to the hundreds of thousands of men with prostate cancer is one way of making up the initial outlay.

CYBERKNIFE

The CyberKnife is not a knife at all but rather a new way of giving radiation therapy to the prostate. This treatment comprises radiation beams that are produced out of a very small linear accelerator as in traditional radiation therapy, as well as a special camera that tracks the movement and position of the prostate during and between treatments.[13] So it is basically a more accurate way of doing radiation therapy but one that requires a general anesthetic, hospitalization, and a catheter for one to two days.[14] None of these is necessary with traditional external beam radiation therapy. And of all these will involve cost to the patient, both in terms of money and convenience.

Like proton beam therapy, this procedure has been used on thousands of patients without the studies to show whether it is of significant benefit. Studies that have been done have focused on safety (yes, it is safe) and different doses of radiation, but it has not gone head to head in studies with other kinds of radiation therapy. Most studies using this technology are very small (under three hundred patients) and suggest that patients experience the same kinds of side effects as with traditional radiation therapy (urinary, bowel, and erectile changes).[15]

There are almost one hundred centers in the United States that have this technology, and it is used to treat other kinds of cancers. It is a treatment that is also advertised widely in an attempt to attract new patients. So the guinea pig issue is pertinent to this treatment as well. We will talk more about this in the chapter on clinical trials (chapter 10).

LIGHT THERAPY (PHOTOTHERAPY)

Phototherapy (or light therapy) is a very new and still experimental treatment for prostate cancer. This treatment involves injecting the man with a drug that is sensitive to light which travels to the prostate gland. Very thin fibers are inserted into the prostate, and these emit light of a specific wavelength that interacts with the drug in the presence of oxygen, causing tissue death. Most of the trials to date involve small numbers of men who had radiation therapy first and then experienced a recurrence of their cancer. There are some studies looking at this as a primary treatment, also with very small numbers of participants.[16]

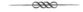

Rod spent most of his days now on the computer. Sue, his wife, found this faintly amusing seeing that he used to shout at her whenever she went on to check e-mail or find a new recipe. Rod just wasn't one for the Internet and computers—that is, until he was diagnosed with prostate cancer.

And then he started to make long-distance calls—even some to England that she only found out about when the phone bill arrived. When he eventually told her what the calls were about, she was speechless—why would he even think about something like this? He showed her the websites that he had been looking at, and he'd even gone to the medical college library where someone had helped him print a stack of papers that she couldn't understand.

And then one day he told her that he'd found out that there was a study at a hospital five hours away and he was going there, with or without her, and he was going to enroll in the study. She was speechless once again. What had happened to her sensible and rational husband who never took any risks?

It's too early to say how effective this treatment is or even to identify with any kind of certainty what the side effects are or will be. In the studies that have been conducted, men experienced urinary problems, but these may have been a result of trauma to the prostate when the fibers were inserted, similar to what happens to men after brachytherapy.[17] An advantage of this procedure is that it can be given more than once if all the cancer is not destroyed, and it can also be given as an out-patient procedure.[18] At the present time, the only way to be able to have this therapy is to be part of a clinical trial; more about that in chapter 10.

WHAT ABOUT HEALTH BEHAVIORS?

We know that the diagnosis of cancer is often a springboard for changes in diet and exercise and other lifestyle factors such as smoking and alcohol intake. Motivation to live a healthier life is high after the shock of diagnosis, and it also gives people something that they can do to have some sort of control in an otherwise uncontrollable situation. So what do we know about health behaviors in men diagnosed with prostate cancer?

Diet

Diet is a topic that the partners/spouses of men with prostate cancer always ask me about. If he eats X and Y and less of Z, will that affect his progress in any way? Can a change in diet cure the cancer? My first response to these questions is clear: a change in diet or taking herbal supplements will *not* cure cancer. That is important information because some men will avoid traditional treatments in favor of something "natural" that is unproven, and the results can be and often are very bad for the patient. Most studies of diet and prostate cancer have focused on prostate cancer prevention, not on disease progression. But there are certain things that the man can do to increase his chances of avoiding progression of his cancer after treatment.

The first is maintaining a healthy weight. Men who are overweight when they have treatment have poorer outcomes, and if they remain overweight after treatment, their risk of having poorer outcomes is increased. We are not sure why this happens, but the evidence is clear: body weight plays a role in progression of prostate cancer, and it also affects quality of life.[19]

The American Cancer Society recommends the following tips for healthy eating for cancer survivors:

- Check with your doctor for any food or diet restrictions.
- Ask your dietitian to help you create a nutritious, balanced eating plan.
- Choose a variety of foods from all the food groups. Try to eat at least five to seven servings a day of fruits and vegetables, including citrus fruits and dark-green and deep-yellow vegetables.
- Eat plenty of high-fiber foods, like whole-grain breads and cereals.
- Buy a new fruit, vegetable, low-fat food, or whole-grain product each time you shop for groceries.
- Decrease the amount of fat in your meals by baking or broiling foods.
- Choose low-fat milk and dairy products.
- Limit salt-cured, smoked, and pickled foods.
- If you choose to drink alcohol, limit the amount.
- If you are overweight, consider losing weight by cutting calories and increasing your activity. Choose activities that you enjoy. Check with your doctor before starting any exercise program.

This information is available on their website: http://www.cancer.org.

They also have an extensive section on exercise and supplements for cancer survivors. These suggestions for healthy eating are much the same as what is generally regarded as a "heart-healthy" diet. The Mayo Clinic website has a good explanation of what comprises a heart-healthy diet. It can be found at: http://www.mayoclinic.com/health/heart-healthy-diet/NU00196.

1. Limit unhealthy fats and cholesterol.
2. Choose low-fat protein sources.
3. Eat more vegetables and fruits.
4. Select whole grains.

5. Reduce the sodium in your food.
6. Control your portion size.
7. Plan ahead: create daily menus.
8. Allow yourself an occasional treat.

Bernie had always had a positive outlook on life, and his wife Rene was not surprised when he told her that he was going to try and take care of the prostate cancer himself before having any kind of surgery or radiation. She knew there was no point in trying to make him change his mind—he was a very stubborn man—and so she asked him just one thing. She wanted him to go to the new center that had opened near where their daughter and son-in-law lived to seek some advice. It was called the Center for Integrative Medicine; her friend Ruth had gone there when she was diagnosed with fibromyalgia, and she couldn't stop talking about how wonderful they were.

Bernie agreed, and Rene went with him to the appointment. They were there for about two hours the first time, and she was most impressed by what they had to say. Bernie seemed less happy—he thought he could just cut down on the beer and the peanuts and take a few vitamins and that would be that. What the staff at the center had in mind was a lot more than that—they wanted him to eat more fruits and vegetables and stop his daily meat and potatoes. And they wanted him to exercise every day! She knew it wasn't kind of her, but she couldn't help smiling in the car on the way home. She'd been saying the same thing for years, and he'd never taken notice. Maybe he would now . . . but only time would tell.

Studies suggest that men with cancer can and do change their dietary habits, often by eating more vegetables, decreasing the amount of fat they eat, and increasing their intake of antioxidants.[20] A similar study showed that changes in diet (increased vegetable intake, decreased animal fat and dairy products) resulted in a lengthening of the time that it took for PSA levels to double.[21] While these were both small, pilot studies, their results are encouraging, especially because the intervention follows the recommendations for a heart-healthy diet.

But is it easy to change one's diet? Many of us know all too well how difficult it is to do this. What we eat is often highly influenced by past patterns (and what we enjoy!), ethnicity, and gender. Male cancer survivors have been shown to have more difficulty or reluctance sticking to a new way of eating than female cancer survivors.[22] So, can you as the partner influence his food choices? Well, that depends. A study from Sweden suggests that female partners positively influence men's food habits,[23] but then another study from the United States has refuted that.[24] A more recent study comparing white and African American men with prostate cancer found that 58 percent had improved their diet by eating more fruits and vegetables and less fat; African American men had made more changes than their white counterparts. Physician recommendation and family support were stated as being of great importance in making these changes.[25]

There is limited evidence on what partners can do to help men make changes to their diet, but if you are the one who controls food shopping and cooking, then you may be able to support a change in his diet by limiting his choices. And a heart-healthy diet is healthy for you too! Of course he can go off by himself and buy whatever he wants, but how likely is he to do this on a daily basis? The 90/10 or 80/20 rule may apply here—eat healthily 80 or 90 percent of the time, and be less strict for the other 10 or 20 percent of the time.

Vitamins, Minerals, and Other Supplements

Men with prostate cancer are known to use complementary medicine; in an Austrian study, one-third of men surveyed used selenium and/or vitamin E, and those who experienced disease progression and poorer quality of life were more likely to use this form of treatment.[26]

Vitamin E, selenium, and lycopene are the most commonly mentioned in the area of prostate cancer, but the important thing to remember is that these have not been shown to play a role in prostate cancer *prevention*, and they do not appear to have a role in prostate cancer progression. There was a lot of publicity about the role of these three substances when trials were started, but unfortunately their lack of effectiveness in preventing prostate cancer has not been widely reported. Many people assume that if something is good for prevention, then it is also good for preventing progression in men with prostate cancer. In the case of vitamin E, selenium, and lycopene, this is not true, and just because something is "natural" does not mean that it won't cause harm. At best taking a vitamin or supplement will be bad for your bank balance, but we do know that vitamin E has been implicated in the deaths of men taking this vitamin, and it may interfere adversely with radiation therapy.[27]

A review by the World Cancer Research Fund and American Institute for Cancer Research states that supplements such as vitamins B, C, and E and selenium are not beneficial to cancer survivors.[28] Experts agree that eating whole foods is always better than supplementing the diet, which once again suggests that following a heart-healthy diet with its emphasis on fruits and vegetables, low-fat protein, and whole grains is the safest and best path to choose.

WHAT COMES NEXT . . .

This chapter discussed newer and experimental therapies for prostate cancer as well as lifestyle changes that may help to avoid disease progression after definitive therapy. But what happens if the cancer does come back? How do you know that a recurrence has occurred, and how do you deal with your feelings if and when it happens? The next chapter will discuss prostate cancer recurrence and further treatment.

What Does This Mean?

Cancer Recurrence

*W*hat happens if the cancer returns after primary treatment? Adjunct (additional) treatment is described in this chapter, as well as the role of chemotherapy that is used for men whose cancer continues to grow despite being starved of testosterone. Recurrence of cancer can be very difficult to deal with, as this may mean that the man will die of his disease. This sensitive topic will be explored in this chapter with suggestions for maintaining hope when things are going wrong.

All men diagnosed with prostate cancer who receive treatment in the form of radical prostatectomy or radiation therapy will be followed for many years by their treating physician or a primary care provider such as a family physician or nurse practitioner. An integral part of this follow-up is regular measurement of the man's PSA level. But why would you measure PSA if the prostate has been removed or irradiated? That's a good question, and the answer will explain a lot about the recurrence of prostate cancer. If you recall the explanation of PSA in chapter 1, you will know that PSA is produced by the prostate gland, so if the prostate gland is no longer there or has essentially been destroyed by radiation, there should be no PSA. Bingo! That is exactly the point: after treatment, the PSA should be at or very near zero. We call this the "PSA nadir"; it is the lowest level that the PSA drops to after treatment. Any change in that number—that is, if the PSA starts to go up—is an indication that the cancer was not completely removed or destroyed; this is called a biochemical recurrence. A measurable PSA level after treatment can also mean that there was some normal prostate tissue left behind that is producing PSA. If you're confused, you're not alone! Even many prostate cancer experts can't agree on exactly what level of PSA indicates that a biochemical recurrence has occurred. Most recurrence is found by a rising PSA, not by any symptoms. Of course if the man does not have follow-up care and the cancer progresses, he may start to have symptoms that suggest the cancer has spread.

Archie was in his early seventies when he was diagnosed with prostate cancer. He had radiation therapy, and everything seemed to be fine. He didn't talk much about it, not even to Rose, his wife, who used to be a nurse. She found this very annoying, but there wasn't much she could do about it. She was more than a little shocked when she answered the phone one day and it was the cancer doctor's office asking why Archie had not been to his scheduled appointment. Why had he missed an appointment? Why did he need an appointment? What was going on?

Archie was not happy with the third degree he got from her when he got home. He vaguely recalled that someone had told him he needed to see the doctor again, but he thought this was a load of nonsense. And old Doc Brewer had told him at a Rotary meeting that he needed to do something or other about having another blood test, but frankly he couldn't be bothered. He just wanted to get on with his life and forget all about the cancer stuff. But Rose had done some reading on the Internet, and she insisted that he go see Dr. Brewer and get his PSA measured. And she didn't let up until he agreed. But he didn't go willingly, and he waited a good three weeks before she dragged him off. He mostly did it to get her off his back. He had no time for doctors but even less time for nagging.

WHAT IS A BIOCHEMICAL RECURRENCE?

A biochemical recurrence is the very earliest sign of treatment failure and is suggested by a PSA level on one or more tests that is higher than zero. It occurs about seven to ten years before the cancer spreads to other organs (usually bone) and about fifteen years before death from prostate cancer.[1] For this reason, treatment of the recurrence is usually started when the doctor sees that the PSA is rising after treatment in order to prevent spreading to other organs and death. Not all men who experience biochemical recurrence will die of prostate cancer. A slowly rising PSA may pose little threat to the man's life—however it may affect his psychological health—and yours as well. Most men diagnosed with prostate cancer are in their sixties or seventies, and so something that may happen fifteen years in the future is not seen as a threat to survival because the man is likely to die of something other than prostate cancer.

Careful monitoring of rising PSA levels after any treatment is complex; it is not just the measurements that are taken into account but also the speed with which the PSA rises. You may hear doctors talking about "PSA doubling times" (how long it takes for the PSA to double) or "PSA kinetics" (PSA values over time and how quickly or slowly they rise). The characteristics of the cancer before treatment, such as the Gleason score and the volume of disease (how many samples from the biopsy had cancer or what volume of the prostate containing cancer was seen after surgery), are also taken into consideration when deciding on future treatment.

RECURRENCE AFTER PROSTATECTOMY

Greg had not worried a bit about what would happen when he was diagnosed with prostate cancer. He was a "get it done" kind of guy, and this philosophy guided his professional and personal life. He didn't want to hear about any treatment other than surgery, and he had his surgery done just one week after his diagnosis. He recovered quickly and has not let anything slow him down, not even the fact that he needs to wear a pad when he exercises. He even told his wife Adrienne that she didn't need to go with him to his follow-up appointments; they were just "routine" according to him, and he wasn't sure why he needed to go so often.

Adrienne was shocked when he called her cell phone the afternoon he went for his checkup; it was eighteen months since the surgery, and she assumed that everything would be fine. She could tell from his voice that something bad had happened; but he wouldn't talk about it on the phone, so she cut short her grocery shopping and hurried home. He was sitting at the dining room table, some papers lying in front of him.

"The cancer's back," he told her in a voice that was shaky.

"What do you mean? Your prostate is gone. . . . How could it be back?" Adrienne realized that she sounded stupid.

"Well, that's as may be. But my PSA has jumped up to two from zero and now I have to have more treatment, and I don't know I can do that . . ."

Adrienne was about to tell him that if he needed more treatment then he had to have it. But she stopped the words from leaving her mouth and instead put her hand on his shoulder. It was going to be a long night for them both.

One-third of men who have had a radical prostatectomy will develop biochemical recurrence within ten years of the surgery.[2] This may be surprising to you because often people assume that if you remove the prostate then there is no risk of the cancer coming back.

If the PSA never goes down to zero or if it starts to rise, the physician has to figure out if the recurrence is local (where the prostate used to be) or if it is distant (spread to the lymph nodes or beyond), or if the PSA level is due to normal prostate tissue at the operative site—or some combination of the three. And to add to the confusion, the PSA value at which there is assurance that this is really a recurrence is controversial among urologists.

The urologist will watch the PSA very carefully if the pathology results from the surgery show that the cancer had spread to the seminal vesicles, if there was extensive cancer that had extended outside the capsule of the prostate gland, or if there were positive surgical margins (evidence of cancer very close to the edges where the cuts were made to remove the gland during surgery). Any of these factors increases the risk of recurrence after surgery.[3]

A stable (but greater than zero) PSA after prostatectomy is most likely due to prostate tissue left behind that continues to produce PSA. A PSA level that reaches 0.2 ng/ml or higher with a subsequent PSA of more than 0.2 ng/ml is regarded as evidence of biochemical recurrence according to the American Urological Society. Other professional bodies use a PSA value of 0.4 ng/ml, which means that different doctors may make different recommendations.

So what should be done about a recurrence? The only treatment that will cure prostate cancer recurrence is radiation therapy to the prostate bed (where the prostate used to be), but this is only useful if the cancer has not spread to the lymph nodes or bones. Finding out this information is more difficult than you would think. Standard tests like CT scans and X-rays do not show where the recurrence is. Whole body scans are also not useful, but a special MRI using a coil in the rectum looks promising for detection of local recurrence in men with a rising PSA level. Bone scans are able to show if the cancer has spread to the bones, and in this case, radiation will not be given; instead the man will receive androgen deprivation therapy (sometimes called hormone therapy). This will be discussed in greater detail in chapter 9.

Radiation therapy after recurrence (also called salvage radiation) cures the cancer in 72 to 90 percent of men and is well tolerated by most men.[4] The duration of treatment is similar to what happens when radiation therapy is used as the primary treatment, and the side effects are also the same.

The addition of androgen deprivation therapy (ADT) to salvage radiation therapy remains controversial. The rationale for this addition is that it is difficult to be completely sure that the cancer has not spread to the lymph nodes and beyond (that is, distant spreading), and so ADT provides extra assurance that the cancer is being treated. But ADT is expensive and has significant side effects as you will read in the following chapter.

RECURRENCE AFTER RADIATION THERAPY

It is estimated that up to 10 percent of men with low-risk prostate cancer (PSA less than 10 and a Gleason score less than or equal to 6, with a normal digital rectal exam) will have a recurrence after radiation therapy. Those with high-risk disease are at much greater risk, up to 60 percent in some studies.[5] A recurrence is said to occur when the PSA level rises by more than 2 ng/ml above the posttreatment PSA. Remember that in men who have radiation therapy, the PSA may never go down to zero because there is still some prostate tissue in the body.

As with recurrence after surgery, difficulties exist in establishing whether the recurrence is local (in the prostate) or distant (lymph nodes or other organs). There are currently no reliable tests to determine the site of recurrence, although MRI is increasingly being used in men with suspicion of recurrence after radiation therapy. In addition, a prostate biopsy after radiation therapy may be performed to prove that there is still cancer in the prostate gland.[6]

So what can be done for men who experience a recurrence after radiation therapy? Quite a lot, actually. Any treatment given for a recurrence is termed "salvage" therapy. I know that this sounds negative (*salvage* means to rescue), but it is a helpful term for medical staff who will know instantly that this is the second line of treatment. The salvage treatment with the longest history is surgical removal of the prostate after the man has been treated with radiation. Sounds simple, doesn't it? If the cancer comes back after radiation, then just take out the prostate and the problem is solved. But it's not that simple. Salvage prostatectomy is a technically difficult procedure with a very high complication rate, which translates into poor quality of life for the man, and also for his partner/spouse. Because of scar tissue that occurs after radiation, the surgery is challenging, and there is a high risk of injury to the rectum, incontinence, and narrowing of the urethra (stricture formation). Erectile problems are also very common.[7] One of the biggest challenges is finding a surgeon who does salvage prostatectomy and who has a lot of experience with this surgery, which will improve outcomes. It is thought that with the newer, more accurate forms of radiation therapy such as 3D-conformal RT, surgery will be easier to perform.[8]

Cryotherapy as described earlier in this book (chapter 7) has been used successfully to treat recurrence after radiation therapy. The same side effects occur when used for recurrence, but recent studies suggest that incontinence occurs in less than 10 percent of men, and general quality of life is satisfactory for most men.[9]

Brachytherapy has also been tried as a salvage therapy, and despite some challenges due to the technical difficulties of inserting seeds into a small gland after radiation, it is considered an appropriate treatment for some men. Studies of brachytherapy as salvage treatment are small with limited postprocedure follow-up.[10]

High-intensity focused ultrasound (HIFU), which you read about in the previous chapter, is also seen as a promising salvage treatment. A small number of studies with limited numbers of patients have shown this to be safe and well tolerated, but further research is needed to determine if this is a viable option for men.[11]

Nothing has gone right for Charles in the past two years. First he found out he had prostate cancer, and just two weeks later his beloved wife was diagnosed with breast cancer. It didn't look good for her—the cancer had already spread to her liver—and so he opted for radiation therapy because then he could take care of her. She died almost six months to the day after her diagnosis; she just seemed to give up hope, and then she was gone. He had just finished his radiation treatments before she became bedridden, and he couldn't remember much of those dark days. He mostly stayed home and thought about how it would have been better if he'd gone first.

He ignored the pain in his right hip that started about two months ago. Just old age, he reckoned. Then one day he fell on the icy path leading up to the house, and when the doctors read his chart they ordered all kinds of tests and then one of them came and told him that the cancer had spread to his bones.

He didn't listen much after that; he really didn't care. When he tried to remember what they'd said, it was mostly just "blah, blah, blah." He and Betty had never had children, so what was the point in having more treatment? He'd rather just let the cancer take its course, and one day, soon he hoped, he'd join Betty in a better place.

The addition of androgen deprivation to any and all of these salvage therapies remains controversial, just as it does with salvage therapy after prostatectomy. Androgen deprivation is not regarded as a cure but will slow down the progression of the cancer. It may be helpful with older men who have limited years of life left, but because of its side effects, it should be used with caution in younger men (see the following chapter for greater detail).[12]

WHAT ELSE CAN HELP?

There is a great deal of interest from physicians as well as men with prostate cancer and their families in alternative treatments for prostate cancer recurrence. Because salvage radiation and androgen deprivation therapy have significant side effects, finding less harmful treatments would pose a significant benefit to these men.

Wally did not think much about traditional medicine. Both of his parents had died of cancer, and this was proof to him that it didn't work. His wife Noreen was a dentist, but they had agreed to disagree on his views many years ago. When she forced him to seek a medical opinion about his nighttime bladder "issues," it started a cascade of blood tests and then a biopsy and then a diagnosis of prostate cancer. Wally flatly refused treatment, but Noreen persuaded him to try his own way (herbs and vitamin C infusions) for six months, and if that got rid of the cancer (she knew it wouldn't), then he wouldn't need further treatment. But if the cancer was still there, he promised he would do something about it.

The herbs and infusions made no difference, so Wally reluctantly agreed to have the seed implant treatment (brachytherapy). When he was done, he started taking a whole collection of herbs. They looked like weeds and sticks to Noreen, but he was convinced that they would keep him healthy. And to keep the peace, Noreen just kept quiet. It was better that way.

Soy has been shown to slow down the rise in PSA in a very small study of men who had been treated with either surgery or radiation.[13] Lycopene, found in cooked tomatoes, has also been shown to stabilize PSA.[14]

Another small study of antioxidants found that an eight-ounce glass of pomegranate juice daily slowed down the time that it took PSA to double in men with recurrence after either prostatectomy or radiation therapy.[15] This was also a small study, with only forty-six men enrolled, but a glass of pomegranate juice is both tasty and not expensive and so may be attractive to both men with prostate cancer and their partners.

There are a number of other small studies that have not yet progressed to the stage where they would be seeking men to enroll in larger studies. These include studies of other medications, such as vitamin D, anti-inflammatory medication, and drugs for benign prostate hypertrophy, that may be useful for men with recurrence of their cancer.[16]

Smoking is associated with an increased risk of recurrence. In addition, men who smoke at the time they are diagnosed with prostate cancer are at increased risk of dying of prostate cancer (they are at a 30 percent increased risk) as well as heart disease. Men who quit smoking ten years before diagnosis are at the same low risk for recurrence as men who never smoked.[17] In another study of men with prostate cancer treated with surgery, 34 percent of smokers, 15 percent of former smokers, and 12 percent of men who never smoked experienced recurrence. Men who smoked one year after surgery had a risk of recurrence twice that of those who never smoked.[16]

These are very strong associations; if there is one thing that you can do for your partner/spouse, helping him to quit smoking or stopping him from starting again is a very good place to start. If you smoke, you must stop to help him stop because it is very difficult to quit alone when there is second-hand smoke in the house or car and the many social triggers for smoking still around. And quitting smoking is good for you too!

Obesity is also associated with increased risk of recurrence for men having surgery. And it's not just the man's weight at the time of surgery; men who gained more than five pounds in the year after the surgery had twice the risk of recurrence of men whose weight remained stable after surgery.[19] And here again is somewhere that you as the partner of the man can help. Regular exercise and a diet that is heart healthy can go a long way toward keeping both of you within the normal limits of weight for your age—and decrease his risk of recurrence. It's a win-win scenario for all!

FEAR OF RECURRENCE

For many cancer survivors, the number-one fear after treatment is that the cancer will come back. This fear varies in intensity for all survivors, with some men thinking about it a lot while other men put the experience behind them and don't focus on recurrence at all or only when they have their PSA measured as part of follow-up care (more about this later). Men who know that the pathology report after surgery showed that there were positive margins (cancer close to the edges of the prostate that was removed) appear to experience more fear of recurrence than men with negative surgical margins, and this fear tends to last for many years after treatment.[20]

Fear of recurrence tends to decline with time; however, some men are never able to forget that they had cancer and continue to worry about recurrence long after the time when it is most likely to happen. For those who experience significant fear of recurrence, we know that they have greater distress and adapt less well than those who don't experience significant fear of the cancer coming back. Men who have better physical and mental health after treatment for prostate cancer were shown to have less fear of recurrence in one study.[21] Men who are satisfied with their treatment choice tend to have less fear of recurrence, and conversely, men who are not satisfied with their treatment choice, often because of the side effects, have greater fear of recurrence and experience poorer quality of life.[22]

For some men, fear of recurrence happens shortly before having their PSA measured as part of their follow-up care. They tend to be anxious while they wait to see the doctor and then experience a rapid decline in anxiety once they learn that everything is okay. For other men, their fear is experienced as intrusive thoughts that occur in response to internal cues (a new pain or sensation in the body) or external cues (reading about prostate cancer in the newspaper or hearing about a sports star who has the disease). These intrusive thoughts tend to pop into one's head and may be experienced as worries or obsessions.

Worry is very common after being diagnosed and treated for cancer. It's easy to see how a prostate cancer survivor may worry about what his next PSA measurement might mean; further treatment and disease progression that may lead to death are all possible negative outcomes. Obsessive thoughts are also possible. A man with prostate cancer would be regarded as having obsessive thoughts if he was convinced that the cancer was back despite repeated testing and assurances that everything is fine.[23]

Ray had lived with bipolar disorder almost all his adult life and had been on medications that controlled it for the past fifteen years. Without the medication, his partner Dennis would most likely have left him. And now, despite the medications, he was in a deep and steep spiral of anxiety. Dennis understood why he was like this—he had taken a long time to get over the side effects of the prostate surgery, and those could depress anyone—but he was very hard to live with now. If he wasn't looking up things on the Internet, then he was in front of the mirror, looking and feeling for signs that the cancer was back. Last night Dennis almost told him to stick his head up his behind because that was the only way he'd see if the cancer was really back—but he decided not to because, with Ray, he might just go ahead and do that! Dennis had explained over and over that Ray's PSA was normal and that Dr. Benson had found nothing wrong on examination, but it made no difference to Ray. Dennis found it frustrating and pathetic, and he was just about out of

patience. You'd think that a gay man who had seen so many friends die of AIDS in the eighties would be grateful for his health and his successful treatment, but not Ray. Dennis was not sure how much more of this he could take.

Living with a man who is experiencing worry, anxiety, and intrusive thoughts can be challenging. There are times when worry and anxiety are appropriate; if his PSA is rising, he may well have cause for concern. But if he worries despite assurances from his health-care providers that there is no evidence of recurrence, nothing you say or do will change that. Irrational worries are just that—irrational—and they don't respond to rational arguments. Supportive counseling may be the best thing for this kind of problem. It may not take the obsessive worrying away, but it can teach him ways to cope with it and may be useful to you too as you learn to cope with his behavior, which no doubt affects you as well.

We don't know much about how the partner/spouse or other close family members experience this fear of recurrence. While we know that spouses of men diagnosed with prostate cancer experience high levels of distress at the time of the diagnosis, little is known about what happens after treatment. Personality type may influence this; if you are a worrier, you may experience more anxiety afterward, and conversely, if you are an optimist, you will likely retain your positive outlook and not worry at all as time goes by.

WHAT COMES NEXT . . .

As promised in this chapter, you will next learn about androgen deprivation therapy and the role it plays in treating and managing prostate cancer. This is an important chapter because many men are prescribed this treatment at some point along the cancer journey. It is a treatment that has lots of side effects and many that will directly affect you and your relationship, so take a deep breath and turn the page.

· 9 ·

How Will He Feel?

Androgen Deprivation Therapy

$\mathscr{P}$rostate cancer is dependent on the male sex hormone testosterone to survive. Preventing the body from producing testosterone is one strategy in the treatment of older men who cannot have surgery or for men with aggressive prostate cancer. But this treatment has profound side effects that will be described in this chapter along with tips and strategies for the spouse/partner for dealing with the fallout from these side effects.

Despite the outlook for many men diagnosed and treated for early prostate cancer that is confined to the gland and has not spread, some men will be diagnosed with high-risk prostate cancer (Gleason score of 8 or above; PSA over 20), or with cancer that has already spread outside the prostate and perhaps even into the lymph nodes or to the bones. Some of these men may not benefit from surgery or radiation because the cancer is outside the prostate. Other men may experience a recurrence of the cancer after surgery or radiation and will need additional treatment. These men are said to have "advanced prostate cancer"; this is a term you will see used over and over in this chapter.

THE TESTOSTERONE CONNECTION

Why do some men have advanced prostate cancer while others are diagnosed with low-risk disease that doesn't pose a risk to their life? There is no simple answer to this question. Some men are diagnosed late in the disease process because they never had a PSA test done and they never had a digital rectal examination; these men may be diagnosed when they have difficulty passing urine and further testing shows the presence of prostate cancer. Other men have aggressive cancer that grows rapidly despite surgery or radiation. Still other men are diagnosed late in life (in their eighties or even nineties) when they experience a broken rib or hip and it is discovered that the fracture was caused by cancer in the bones that originated in the prostate. It is difficult at any time to be diagnosed with cancer, but when the prognosis is uncertain, many couples find that the shock of diagnosis is compounded by the very real threat to life.[1] This also flies in the face of the very many men who are diagnosed with low- or intermediate-risk cancer whose lives are not compromised by the cancer and who fall into the group of men who will die *with* prostate cancer, not of it.

Thomas thought he'd done everything right—he was not overweight, he exercised regularly, he watched how much he drank—so when he was told he had high-risk prostate cancer, he just couldn't believe it. His wife Mary took the news really badly; he came from a family where most everyone lived well into their nineties, so how could this happen to him? She raged against the news, and at times Thomas felt like she was angry with him. She buried herself in articles she found on the Internet, and she badgered his doctor with her questions. Thomas could see that the urologist was getting irritated with her demands, but frankly, he was so shocked himself that he just let her do what she felt she needed to. It didn't help when the urologist said that Thomas was beyond being helped by surgery. At this news, Mary went wild! She cried and screamed at the urologist to the point that he had to call his assistant in to calm her down. Thomas just didn't have the strength to stop her or support her. He just watched her implode, and part of him wished he could just let go like that.

An important fact to know about this situation is that when the cancer has gone outside the gland itself, the focus on treatment changes from cure to control. This can be something that is very difficult to accept; the good news is that the cancer can be controlled in some men for many years. The bad news is that eventually the cancer will become resistant to this control, and the man may die of prostate cancer.

For these men the only treatment option left is to deprive the cancer of its fuel, the male hormone (sometimes called an "androgen") testosterone. Here's a short biology lesson: Testosterone is the hormone that causes the characteristic changes when a boy becomes a man. Body and facial hair, growth of the penis and testicles, widening of the shoulders and increased muscle growth and strength, deepening of the voice, sexual interest (libido), and erections are all a product of testosterone. Testosterone is produced by the testicles (and to a much lesser extent by the adrenal glands that sit on top of the kidneys) under the influence of messages from the brain. The prostate gland itself contains androgen receptors that respond to the presence of testosterone and signal the cells in the gland to grow. Androgen receptors also instruct the prostate to produce PSA, so when you shut down testosterone production in the testicles (more about this later), you also shut down these receptors, and PSA stops being produced. This is important for you to know because understanding the role of testosterone and androgen receptors will help you to understand the rest of this chapter. The biology lesson is now over!

WHAT IS THE TREATMENT FOR A MAN WITH ADVANCED PROSTATE CANCER?

This is one of those questions that has an "it depends" answer. Treatment options are based on the extent of the cancer, its rate of growth (measured by how quickly or slowly the PSA is rising), as well as the man's age, general health, and his (and your) willingness to accept the risks of treatment. More about this later.

One option is to *watch what happens over time* (watchful waiting) and only treat symptoms as they occur. This may be a reasonable option for a man whose PSA is rising slowly and who has no evidence of metastatic spread (for example to the bones). Because there is no cure for men with advanced disease, the goal of treatment is to help him live as well as possible, and that means controlling any symptoms when they occur and not causing him any treatment-related suffering from side effects. If cancer has spread to the bones, radiation therapy directed at the places where the cancer has settled can provide great relief from pain and reduce the risk of fracture. This form of radiation is given over a couple of days and does not have the same sorts of risk for side effects that you have read about when radiation is given to the prostate gland with the intent to cure the cancer.

The medical team will monitor his PSA regularly and may order other tests (such as an MRI and bone scan) every year. They will focus particularly on the PSA doubling time; the time (in months or years) that it takes for the PSA to double is a valuable indicator of cancer growth. A PSA doubling time of more than a year is a good sign as is a PSA that does not rise above 20. Many men with advanced prostate cancer can live with a slowly rising PSA and no other symptoms of spread for many years.

Androgen deprivation therapy (ADT) has become the mainstay of treatment for advanced prostate cancer. In 1941, Dr. Charles Huggins discovered that prostate cancer was dependent on testosterone for continued growth; he was awarded the Nobel Prize for his work. He showed that by removing a man's testicles, or giving him the female hormone estrogen, testosterone production was stopped, and men with spread to the bones almost miraculously recovered and were able to resume their lives. It is important to remember that this is not a curative treatment but rather palliative (controlling symptoms), and most men experience a return of the prostate cancer because the cancer learns to survive and grow without the fuel of testosterone.

ADT is often called "hormone therapy." I prefer to not use this term because it implies that we are giving the man hormones (much like some women are given hormones during and after menopause). What we do is deprive men of their androgens (testosterone), and I believe that by being accurate in naming this treatment, we make ourselves aware of the state of hormonal deprivation men experience.

Chuck—or Charles, as his wife Emily calls him—has been living with prostate cancer for almost five years. He was diagnosed on his seventy-fifth birthday, and he knew that this was going to happen—three of his four brothers had "prostate troubles," so in a way he had been waiting for this. The last five years have not been easy for him, and especially not for Emily, who has had to take care of him. Chuck has never taken good care of himself, and now at eighty he feels like a very old man. He has bad arthritis in his hips and knees, and on top of the cancer, he has heart problems. He's been offered surgery for that—but he has never been convinced that going under the knife is a solution for anything. So with the bad hips and knees, and the fatigue from his heart condition, he doesn't go out much or do much of anything. Emily has had to do everything around the house, and while she says she's okay with that, there are times when she is irritable with him.

And now the doctor has told him that he needs to do something about the cancer—the tests show that it's growing, and they're suggesting that he either have his testicles removed or he can have these injections. Imagine! Cutting a man's manhood off—Chuck is not having any of that! So he tells Emily that he has to go back to the doctor for injections every three months—and when she finds out how much they cost, she tells him that she'll cut off his testicles and then he'll be done. That shocked him to the core—why would she say that?

Androgen deprivation can be achieved in a couple of different ways. The first is to remove the testicles; the medical term for this is *orchiectomy*. This used to be the only way to stop testosterone production, but it is not done all that often now, mostly because men are no longer offered this option since the introduction of medication (in the form of injections) to halt production. It is thought that men find the idea of removal of the testicles (surgical castration) to be psychologically difficult. It is a simple surgery to perform with few side effects, and the surgeon can put in testicular implants that feel very much like the real thing. I have spoken to men who were never offered the option of this surgery, and they have told me that if they'd known about it, they would have preferred this to the injections (and their cost!).

The second and most popular form of ADT is medication given in the form of injections (every one, three, four, six, or even twelve months). These are called LHRH agonists, and the way they act is by interfering with a signal from the brain to the testicles to produce testosterone. These drugs are known by the trade names Leupron, Eligard, Zoladex, Vantas, or Decapeptyl. Initially the body responds to the rapid drop in testosterone levels by trying to increase testosterone production (this is called a testosterone flare), so most men are also prescribed another medication for a short time (called an anti-androgen) to control this increase.

Antiandrogens (called Casodex or Nilandron) are often used with LHRH agonists—this is called a complete or total androgen blockade. They do not seem to add any advantage after the first few weeks when they control the testosterone flare, and they do add side effects, so they are usually not used beyond the first couple of weeks. They do not have a role to play in men who have had an orchiectomy.

Some studies have suggested that antiandrogens alone (without LHRH agonists) can be useful for men with advanced prostate cancer and may avoid some of the sexual side effects that you will read about later in this chapter. It should be noted that the higher doses of these drugs that need to be used when an antiandrogen is given alone are not approved by the FDA and are used as an off-label treatment. Men with metastatic disease should not use this form of therapy and should be on LHRH agonists.

WHEN SHOULD ADT BE STARTED?

This is a hotly debated topic in cancer circles, and opinions seem to outweigh the evidence. The jury is out on when a man should start ADT in any form, with some experts saying that earlier is better, while others suggest that waiting until later reduces the risk of side effects.[2] Part of the issue is that there haven't been a lot of studies to provide evidence of the usefulness of starting the treatment as soon as the PSA starts to rise, so many physicians have their own opinions on the matter and practice accordingly. In addition, some men may pressure their physicians to "do something" when the PSA starts to rise. Starting ADT early has not been shown to extend life expectancy, and it has significant side effects.[3] After reading the next section on the side effects of ADT, you may have your own opinion to add to this debate.

There is another debate on this topic too: should ADT be given continuously or should the man be allowed to stop it when the PSA drops and then restart only when it goes up again? This second regimen is called "intermittent ADT." There is increasing evidence that this approach may be useful in some men, primarily those with advanced disease who do *not* have metastatic disease. So it may be appropriate for those men who want to start doing something earlier rather than later. One of the very real advantages of intermittent therapy is that it reduces the side effects and allows the man to spend 30 to 50 percent of his remaining life without these side effects (or with limited side effects) and so with better quality of life. The man needs to be closely monitored (PSA and testosterone levels) for signs of disease progression and the treatment started again at the earliest sign of any change.[4]

Jacques (Jim to his friends) has had a hard time adapting to the changes he's experienced since being on the injections. He's had every side effect in the book—hot flashes that wake him and his partner Joe, irritability, forgetfulness, and of course his sex life has gone down the tubes faster than a greased hog. He asked his doctor if he could stop, and the response was, "If you want to die, you can." This did not sit right with Jacques, so he spent some time in the medical library, and he found out that some doctors let their patients have a drug vacation. Once again he approached his doctor, this time with a binder full of articles from the library, and this time the doctor said he could stop for a while and see what happened to his PSA. Joe had gone with him to that appointment, and Jacques told him that his presence (he was six foot four inches tall and pushing three hundred pounds) had intimidated the doctor. Joe thought it had something to do with the doctor being uncomfortable with their relationship, but he didn't say that to Jacques—what was the point? There were not that many choices when it came to finding a urologist where they lived, and this guy was generally okay. And after all, Jacques had gotten his way—he was going to hopefully get back his energy and libido, and with it his zest for life. So who cares why or how?

WHAT ABOUT USING ADT FOR MEN *WITHOUT* ADVANCED DISEASE?

Despite studies that have shown that using ADT as a primary treatment for men with localized prostate cancer is not a good idea (because of side effects and the risk that the cancer will grow despite the absence of testosterone), this use continues, probably because of anxiety in men and their physicians who don't want to be seen to be "doing nothing." This is especially prevalent in older men who don't need surgery or radiation but are not comfortable with the decision to not treat the cancer. A number of studies have shown that when older men (sixty-five and older) with prostate cancer that has not spread (that is, localized prostate cancer) are treated with ADT, there is no survival benefit,[5] and it may in fact cause worse outcomes for these men than monitoring them closely and not starting ADT.[6]

So why do physicians prescribe this medication for men with localized prostate cancer when there is no evidence to support its use for these men? The numbers of men with localized disease receiving ADT as primary therapy is not insignificant; one survey of practice patterns showed that 14 percent of men with localized disease had been prescribed ADT.[7]

As discussed previously, part of the answer may lie in pressure from patients (and perhaps their partners), who don't want to just wait and see what happens. Another part of the answer may lie in the kind of physician who is caring for the men. One study found that urologists who practiced outside of academic centers, who had graduated less recently, and who had large numbers of patients were more likely to prescribe ADT for patients with localized disease who should not be getting this treatment. In addition, it is well known that there is a financial incentive to use these medications because physicians can purchase them from the pharmaceutical companies at a bulk discount and then charge patients and/or their insurance carriers for the treatment, usually at a profit.[8] Since the introduction of LHRH agonists in the 1980s, the use of these medications has increased, and the number of orchiectomies has decreased, especially in the Medicare population in the United States. The Medicare Modernization Act (MMA) in 2003 came about as a result of skyrocketing costs for these medications ($1 billion in 2001). Under this act, reimbursement to physicians for Medicare patients was reduced so that by 2005, reimbursement was at 40 to 50 percent of what it had been in 2003. The result of this was a significant decrease in the use of these medications and a rise in the rates of orchiectomy. Of interest is that a new LHRH agonist was not included in the list of medications that were no longer covered at pre-MMA levels; this medication saw an increase in use of 2,786.2 percent during the same time period![9] Coincidence perhaps? I'll let you decide.

SIDE EFFECTS OF ADT

Many men decide on a primary treatment for prostate cancer based on the side-effect profile of each treatment; you have read about these in great detail in the preceding chapters. Men with advanced or metastatic prostate cancer may not have that choice and instead are prescribed ADT, which, while it may lengthen life, comes with a very significant risk of serious side effects. The side effects of ADT can be grouped as follows:

1. Sexual changes
2. Physical changes
3. Metabolic changes
4. Emotional and cognitive changes
5. Quality-of-life changes

The next section of this chapter will describe these changes, how they may affect you, and what if anything you can do to deal with them or help the man cope.

Sexual Changes

One of the biggest and most bothersome changes for most men on ADT is the loss of sexual interest (also called libido) that they experience. This occurs in about 85 to 90 percent of men and is the number-one complaint for my patients. Testosterone is the hormone of desire for men (we're not sure about its role in women), and the sudden and complete drop in testosterone levels is surprising and often devastating for men. In a touching essay published in the *Journal of the American Medical Association*,[10] Dr. Howard Harrod describes what life was like for him without testosterone after his diagnosis of aggressive prostate cancer:

> The sudden loss of libido produced forms of suffering I had not anticipated. . . . I taught at a university each day. . . . I encountered young people caught in the throes of raging hormones. Because I had lost the capacity to experience desire did not mean that I was not tormented by *memories* of desire.

It can be difficult to try to explain what this loss of libido means to men. Perhaps the easiest way to do it is to start with what is normal for most men: men tend to live in a hormonal milieu that is rich in testosterone. This hormone feeds every aspect of their lives, and while there are many jokes about men being totally motivated by sex, the jokes are not far off. That doesn't mean that all men think about sex all the time and act on these thoughts all the time, but sexual desire is part of their everyday existence. Without testosterone, all of this changes. Most men (and there are always exceptions) on ADT stop thinking about sex, stop talking about sex, stop having erotic dreams, and, importantly, stop touching their partners. This is not conscious or intentional; it's as if that part of themselves has just been switched off.

They also are not able to have erections, and the testicles and penis shrink by as much as 25 percent.[11] This lack of erections in addition to lack of desire in turn affects how a man experiences masculinity, and some men no longer regard themselves as a "whole man."[12]

Bob and June used to be the target of their friends' jokes because they were the ones who always held hands, always sat next to each other, and seemed to be constantly touching each other. They'd always been like that through the five years of their courtship and fifty-two years of marriage. But since he went on the injections, it's as if he were a cold, hard piece of stone. She tried talking to him about it, but he just looked at her like she had grown horns out of the top of her head. He didn't seem to understand what the problem was, and she found herself getting angry with him, which surely didn't help as he just withdrew even further.

At first June thought it was her fault—that she wasn't attractive enough, that the fifteen pounds she'd put on after the menopause was the reason. But she'd carried those fifteen pounds for almost ten years now, and they didn't seem to make a difference before. She even thought that maybe he was having an affair, but one night they went to the support group and she heard from some of the other women that the same thing had happened with their husbands. Now they couldn't all be having affairs, could they? The other women described exactly what she had been going through—no touching, no kissing, no cuddling—and while it helped June to know that she was not alone, none of them seemed to have been able to do anything about it.

Now some of you may think that if a man is not able to have erections then not wanting sex may be a good thing. Some men would agree with that statement, but many do not. Men tell me that while their desire and erections may be gone, their memories still remain, and much like the quote from Dr. Harrod above, they remember what life used to be like, and this emphasizes what they have lost. They may avoid their male friends because they are afraid that any talk or joking about sex will shine a spotlight on their inability in this area, and this in turn will lead to them feeling like less of a man, or even to being teased and humiliated by their friends.

Lack of interest in sex can have profound effects on the spouse/partner too. Many couples use sex as their primary way of showing affection, so no sex can mean no other shows of affection either. The partners of men on ADT complain about this all the time to me. They may not miss the sex, but they do miss the touching, holding hands, and those special glances across the room. All of that goes too. This lack of touch is different from the avoidance that some men show when they are unable to have erections after surgery or radiation; these men still feel the need to touch their partner, but when on ADT, it seems that the need for touch goes away.

The effect of lack of libido and profound erectile dysfunction on the relationship between men and their partners has been clearly described in a study from Israel.[13] The men in this study reported a wide-ranging number of losses after they started ADT. They felt that they were no longer "real" men and reported that their wives treated them differently. This loss of their previous masculine role led to depression, feelings of worthlessness, and tension in the relationship. Both the men and their spouses were shocked by the changes these men experienced and seemed unprepared for what life was like while on ADT. In terms of sexuality, some of the couples attempted to maintain a semblance of their patterns before the treatment, but eventually this became burdensome and they stopped trying. For some men in this study, they found that their inability to have erections allowed them to stop bothering their wives for sexual activity, and they were grateful that they did not pressure their wives anymore. Many couples who continue to attempt to keep sexual activity alive in the relationship become frustrated over time, and feelings of doubt and hopelessness are not uncommon.[14]

Some couples seem to fare better. The diagnosis often prompts increased sharing and expressions of love and support between partners. Some men report that being on ADT allows them to express their feelings without the restriction that society places on men (and women) about what is masculine and what is not. Dr. Richard Wassersug has written widely on the topic of what ADT does to masculine self-image and male sexuality, and he suggests that with less emphasis on the penis for sexual expression, there is room for exploration of alternative activities for both partners to experience pleasure in different ways.[15] Some couples are able to maintain and even improve their sexual experiences by focusing on nonpenetrative activities and whole-body sensations.

So what can be done about this lack of libido and inability to have erections? As stated previously, absence of libido may decrease frustration over ED. However, for those men who continue to experience libido, the usual interventions for achieving erections may not be as successful when the man has very low testosterone. Even when the man uses erectile aids (for example medications such as Viagra, Cialis, or Levitra), the chances of success are about 40 percent, and this is in part influenced by age and other medical illnesses.[16]

We often think that if we inform patients and partners of potential side effects, this will help them adapt. This is not always the case, and I have certainly found that couples may have an intellectual understanding of what

ADT can do to their sex life, but the reality is something quite different. The words "He may stop touching you because he just doesn't think about it" are very different from the reality of what living without physical contact of any kind is like. Couples often don't appreciate the role that sex, even if very infrequent, plays in the connection between partners. It can be a challenge for the partner to be the one who initiates touch, especially if it was usually the man who approached the partner. This requires a change in role that is challenging, particularly after years of being the recipient and not the initiator of sexual advances and touch.

In addition, the partner may unconsciously interpret lack of touch or approach as rejection. Relationships are complex and multilayered, and there are hidden meanings and assumptions in many aspects of partnered life. Being able to overcome the challenges of ADT requires communication that is open and honest and descriptive, and many couples find this very difficult. You will read a little later about some of the emotional changes that men experience while on ADT, and this can also have an impact on the couple's ability to talk about sensitive topics without hurt feelings and the fear of causing pain to one's partner.

Loss of libido also takes place at the same time as other side effects that may compound how the man feels about himself. You will read in the next sections about feminization of the body, fatigue, and emotional changes, and these all play a role in his and your sexuality. Simple suggestions (take a pill, talk more, use a prompt [when the news starts on TV] to remind you touch your partner every day) are usually not helpful because they are too simple and don't take into account everything that is going on in your life.

Many couples find a visit to a sex therapist or counselor very helpful. These professionals are experts who can help with suggestions for alternative means of sexual expression, and they can help couples communicate about sensitive issues in a safe and empowering environment.

Physical Changes

Being deprived of testosterone causes physical changes as well. These include having hot flashes, weight gain, breast enlargement and tenderness, loss of muscle mass and strength, and changes in amount and appearance of body hair.

Lionel was not a man who took being sick very well; he'd been healthy all his life and prided himself on never missing a day of work in forty years in his lab. Soon after retiring at seventy-one years of age, he found out he had prostate cancer, and not the good kind either. His wife Maureen and their kids (twin boys aged thirty-seven)

insisted that he go on the injections even though he didn't want to. The worst thing was the sweating. He'd always been one to sweat a lot—when he was younger, he would sweat right through his T-shirt when cutting the grass—but now it was like he was some kind of fountain. He'd suddenly get really hot, and the sweat would just pour off his forehead and drip down his nose. It was embarrassing. He'd be having coffee with the guys, old high school friends who met most mornings at a coffee shop, and suddenly he'd be drenched. At first the guys just ignored it, but he knew it was hard to ignore. Mort asked him one time why he sweating like that—they were just sitting around and shooting the breeze, after all—and then Lionel had to tell them about the cancer and the injections, and he hated to see the look on their faces. He'd always been the strong one—two of them had heart problems, and they'd lost Paulie to lung cancer the year before—so to have to admit to something like cancer was difficult. Now he was the target of their pitiful looks, and he hated it.

One of the earliest and most bothersome physical changes is the occurrence of *hot flashes.* When I talk to couples about this in preparation for the man starting ADT, they often comment that he will now know what his female partner went through during menopause. There is a lot of truth to this; women also experience hot flashes during and after menopause, and most research on this phenomenon has been done with women. Men are different from women in one important aspect: they have many more sweat glands, and so they report a higher intensity of sweating than women do.

Let's talk about what a hot flash feels like (if you need reminding!). Hot flashes are described as a feeling of heat that spreads from the chest to the rest of the body, often accompanied by profuse sweating on the forehead, chest, and back, followed by chills.[17] They can be triggered by a change in temperature in the room, spicy foods, hot liquids, or changes in body position. If mild in intensity, they are usually well tolerated, but if they are moderate to severe, they can be intolerable, and some men find them so bad and their impact on their quality of life so significant that they stop their ADT therapy. They often occur more frequently at night and cause drenching sweats resulting in disturbed sleep. The man often needs to get up and change his bedclothes and sheets, leading to sleep deprivation if this occurs for a long period of time. Sleep deprivation in turn leads to mood changes, difficulty concentrating, and memory problems. And if he's getting up and changing clothes and sheets, then you are too, and that results in two people with sleep deprivation. This is often the reason that partners sleep in separate bedrooms (and the snoring of course!).

While separate bedrooms are very common (and often necessary), this may mean that it takes a fair amount of effort for couples to find time to cuddle and have that "pillow talk" that is so important for intimacy if they are not sleeping in the same bed. If the man is on ADT, the motivation to cuddle may be absent, which puts additional pressure on you to initiate and maintain touch. Another challenge for you!

Hot flashes are reported by 34 to 80 percent of men on ADT, and almost a third say they are the most troublesome side effect of the treatment.[18] They tend to start early after the initiation of therapy and persist for years after treatment. They also serve as a constant reminder of the cancer and contribute to cancer-related distress.[19] They can also affect the man's ability to work and socialize with others. If he is bothered or embarrassed by the hot flashes (turning red in the face and sweating profusely can do this), he may avoid social situations or give up work, leading to social isolation.

What can be done about them? Most of the research on interventions for hot flashes has been done on women, and the results aren't hopeful. Various forms of estrogen have been studied in men, but these have severe side effects, including growth of breast tissue (more about that in the next section of this chapter) and increased risk of blood clots and heart disease. Megestrol acetate also has the risk of severe side effects similar to estrogen. Newer antidepressants such as the selective serotonin reuptake inhibitors (SSRIs) show some promise but also have side effects including sexual dysfunction and weight gain. Gabapentin (Neurontin) is a medication that is used for nerve pain and has shown some promise in treating hot flashes, but no large trials have been done; this medication can also cause significant side effects.

There is great interest in nonhormonal and more natural treatments for hot flashes. Isoflavones from soy products have not shown any effect for men (and mixed results for women).[20] The most hopeful intervention to date is acupuncture, which in one study resulted in a more than 50 percent reduction in 41 percent of the men treated in just four weeks.[21]

Another side effect of ADT is changes to the man's body resulting in altered *body image* and physical strength. Testosterone makes men look like men—broad shoulders, narrow hips, facial and body hair—and without it, changes occur that are often called "feminizing" (making men look like women). This is an inaccurate description, but there are certain physical changes that make men look different than they did before. These include weight gain, loss of muscle mass and strength, changes to body hair, and the development of breasts.

Let's start by talking about *breast enlargement*, which is called "gynecomastia" by medical professionals. It is most often caused by taking an antiandrogen alone; Casodex is the drug that appears to cause this side effect most often. In men taking this drug, almost half will experience breast enlargement, and almost 75 percent will experience pain and tenderness in that area.

This is embarrassing and distressing to many men, and some may avoid social situations because of it or change how they dress to minimize appearance of the breasts. This is not fat but rather growth of glandular tissue as a result of an increased ratio of estrogen to testosterone in the body (yes, men do have estrogen, but it's usually in small amounts). This breast enlargement doesn't go away even if treatment is stopped, although this is more likely to occur if the man has been on the medication for a year or more. It's also quite difficult to treat; the most common treatments are surgery to remove excess tissue or radiation therapy to the area, which is often given at the start of treatment to try and prevent growth of the tissue.[22]

Hugh was at a loss—as a former wrestler he was used to looking a certain way—muscular and manly. But it was as if someone had waved a wand over his body, and it had all turned to fat. He had known it was a possibility; the nurse at the oncologist's office had warned him about it, but he didn't think it would happen to him. He had always been so fit and strong; those hours and hours in the gym, a habit he continued long after his wrestling days were over, had kept him in good shape. He had a new girlfriend, Patricia, and he was now afraid to take off his shirt in front of her. He'd stopped wearing T-shirts completely because of the way he looked in them, like a puffed-up marshmallow; instead he wore big flannel shirts that covered up the rolls of fat. He'd stopped going to the gym because he couldn't wear shorts and a T-shirt anymore—and not exercising made him grumpy. Patricia had commented on his mood yesterday, and he hated to think that he could lose her. But she said he was not the guy she had met, and she looked sad when she said it.

Men on ADT also tend to gain *weight*, particularly in the abdomen. This happens within the first year of treatment and is a source of distress for the men.[23] Weight gain in this area is also associated with something called the "metabolic syndrome," which will be discussed in the next section. It is very frustrating for men, it is hard to get rid of with diet and exercise, and it has a negative impact on quality of life.[24]

Most men on ADT will also experience *changes in hair growth and texture*. Body hair will decrease and become softer, and many men find that they do not have to shave their beards as often. While this may be seen as a bonus by some, others will see this as a reminder of the cancer on a daily basis, and it may also factor into their view of themselves as men or their masculine self-image.

Men also lose muscle mass and strength (up to five pounds in the first year on treatment), which has implications for body image as well as functional ability. A loss of muscle strength can impact his ability to work or do the things that are usually considered part of the male role. More about that later. Loss of muscle mass also contributes to a changed shape (smaller shoulders in contrast to a wider midsection) and may mean that the man has to purchase new clothing. Of particular concern is the increased risk of falls in men with decreased muscle mass, as well as general frailty.

So what can you do to help him cope with these physical changes? It goes without saying that you should be supportive—you wouldn't be reading this book if you weren't!—but there are some practical things you can do as well. Encouraging him to get regular exercise can make him feel better about himself, even if he still hates what he sees in the mirror. We will talk more about the role of exercise in the following pages as it relates to the prevention of bone loss, but exercise is good for the heart, mind, and body. Exercise can help with depression, and it also has a role to play in managing weight gain and bone strength. It is very important that men on ADT do resistance exercise to maintain muscle mass and strength. The most common form of resistance exercise is lifting weights; this should be done under the supervision of a trained professional at a gym or in your home gym. This has financial implications and may not be affordable for everyone. Some men may not want to go to the gym because of their altered shape and weight gain. You can purchase resistance bands at most sporting goods stores; these bands can be used instead of weights, but the man should be taught how to use them properly and safely by a trained professional.

The changes described above are all physical and don't contribute to ill health (other than decreased muscle mass and frailty), but they are distressing. Some men have reported that their partners avoid touching them in response to the changes in their bodies.[25] There are, however, other side effects of ADT that do threaten the man's health and that are serious.

Metabolic Changes

Lack of testosterone is known to affect the bones and cardiac system, putting the man at risk for conditions such as osteoporosis, diabetes, high cholesterol, high blood pressure, and heart disease. Sounds serious? Yes, it is. Age certainly plays a role in the development of these conditions, even in otherwise healthy men, but the ADT seems to hasten or worsen these changes. Most men with prostate cancer are over the age of sixty-five, and many of them will already have some of these conditions.

Osteoporosis is a condition of the bones caused by decreased bone mineral density that puts a person at increased risk of fracture. This is different from the cancer spreading to the bones as discussed earlier in this chapter. Women are also at risk for osteoporosis after menopause as a result of declining estrogen levels, and the same thing happens to men as they age as a result of decreased testosterone levels. It is estimated that 25 to 40 percent of older men have osteoporosis when they are diagnosed with prostate cancer, and then ADT speeds up the decline in bone strength.[26] This bone loss starts within the first few months of taking the medication and is worst in the first year, after which the decrease in bone strength continues but at a slower rate.

It is very important that this decrease in bone strength be monitored closely, starting with a baseline DEXA scan, which should be repeated after one year on ADT. There is debate among medical professionals about the role of bisphosphonate therapy in men at risk for osteoporosis; you have probably seen ads on TV and in magazines for these medications aimed at women after menopause.

It's very important for men on ADT to do weight-bearing exercise on a regular basis to prevent further bone loss (and for heart health, as you'll see shortly). Walking and jogging are examples of weight-bearing exercise, but swimming is not. Resistance exercises are also important. Daily vitamin D and calcium supplements are essential; men should take 1,200 to 1,500 mg of calcium every day and enough vitamin D to keep their blood levels between 50 and 75 mN. There are also things to avoid: smoking and more than two alcoholic drinks per day are known to contribute to bone mineral loss.

Your encouragement and support in helping him maintain a regular exercise schedule may be the tipping point between him getting the exercise he needs and not getting enough. And the same kind of exercise is important for you too—so exercise together, and you'll both see the benefits.

Men on ADT are at increased risk for something called "insulin resistance syndrome" (SupportiveOncology.net). This results in increased insulin levels, obesity, and increased risk of cardiac disease because of raised lipid levels in the blood. These changes start within the first three months of taking ADT and significantly raise the risk for developing *diabetes*. For men who already have diabetes, more aggressive treatment may be necessary to control insulin and glucose levels in the blood. Close monitoring of his glucose levels is important.

The association of *cardiac disease* and ADT is one that is hotly debated in medical journals. Some studies suggest that ADT increases a man's risk of dying from a heart attack or stroke, while other studies show no increased risk. Close control of lipid and cholesterol levels in the blood is important; medication may be needed if diet is not enough. All cardiac risk factors, especially smoking, should be minimized or avoided. Once again, regular exercise (and your encouragement that he do it) can play an important role in controlling weight gain and preventing diabetes. These metabolic changes start within three to six months of starting ADT, so beginning a regular exercise routine should start with the first injection.

Emotional and Cognitive Changes

Sylvia was at her wits' end. Her husband Mark had turned into someone else entirely. When she looked at him she could hardly recognize the man she married so many years ago. He had turned into a crabby old man, and at sixty-eight, he really shouldn't be like that. It had all started when he insisted that Dr. Brownlee start him on those darn injections. Dr. Brownlee didn't think it was necessary, but Mark had made up his mind. He'd been going online for hours at a time after he was diagnosed, and somehow he'd read something there that got him all excited about the injections. Not only were they really expensive, but they had changed him. He didn't sleep well anymore, but it was the mental stuff that she found hardest to take. He was irritable all the time, and not just with her—just this past weekend he had yelled at their grandchildren when they were playing in the study after Sunday brunch. Visits from the grandchildren had always been such a highlight of their week, but last Sunday they left in tears, hustled to the car by their mom, Sandy, their only daughter. Sandy had looked at her mom with tears in her eyes and a question behind the tears—what was up with her dad?

Many men on ADT report mood changes while on treatment; their partners often corroborate these changes. Some of my patients report getting weepy often, where before they were more stoic. Some partners/spouses describe a man who is more sensitive and less "macho" but at the same time more irritable and likely to get annoyed at small things.

The research on this is unclear. Some studies report increased *anxiety and irritability* in men on ADT. One study suggests that these emotional changes go away when the ADT is stopped,[27] but there is also the chance that this is related to the fact that the cancer has progressed rather than to the ADT itself. It may also be related to fatigue (more about that later) and sleep disturbance because of hot flashes.

The incidence of *depression* in men on ADT has also been studied, with conflicting results. Some studies show no increase in depression[28] while others report that men say they are depressed.[29] Once again this may be related to age (most men with advanced prostate cancer are older than those diagnosed with early cancer), other health conditions, or more advanced cancer that requires treatment with ADT.

Some authors have described something called "androgen deprivation syndrome," comprising depression, memory difficulties, and fatigue.[30]

This syndrome has been described in as many as 30 percent of men on ADT, but once again there is some question about the exact cause—the ADT itself, or age, other conditions, or the knowledge of advanced cancer.

Despite what the studies say, what do you do if you think your partner/ spouse is depressed? The answer is simple: get help. His primary care provider has a range of treatment options including antidepressant medications and counseling. As you have read earlier in this book, exercise is an effective way of treating mild to moderate depression, and it has the added benefits discussed at length earlier in this chapter. I know it sounds as if I am selling exercise—but it really works! And if you exercise along with him, you can deal with your own tensions or anxiety from dealing with his illness.

As the partner of a man with prostate cancer on ADT, you will likely be the first to notice changes in *cognitive functioning*. Most commonly seen are changes in spatial abilities (the ability to manipulate two- and three-dimensional figures), which is one area where men traditionally do better than women. Think about putting together a gas barbecue with hundreds of nuts and bolts; spatial ability will help with thinking about how to translate what's on the paper into the action of getting the nuts and bolts in the right place. While you can avoid putting together gas barbecues, men who work in professions where spatial ability is central to their day-to-day activities (e.g., architects, carpenters, construction workers) may face significant challenges in being able to continue working.

Men on ADT also see declines in working memory (the ability to actively hold information in the brain in order to do complex tasks such as reasoning, comprehension, and learning). You may notice this first when he can't remember how to do something like programming the PVR to record his favorite program. Or he may find it difficult to problem solve something new that he has not encountered before. These signs can sometimes be subtle, so you may only recognize them in retrospect.

What can help with these cognitive changes? Besides adapting to the changes for both of you, a referral to an occupational therapist may be helpful. These professionals may be able to help both of you cope with changes and find "work-arounds" to minimize the impact of the changes. You may also find yourself taking up the slack and doing the things that he can't anymore. This may present an interesting challenge to you or be a source of frustration and sorrow when your roles change. It's important to take care of yourself and keep yourself healthy with these challenges, so please make sure that you read chapter 14 about self-care.

Quality-of-Life Changes

Men on ADT also experience lowered levels of hemoglobin in their blood. Hemoglobin is found in red blood cells and is responsible for carrying oxygen to the tissues. Low levels of hemoglobin result in fatigue (anemia—low levels of red blood cells—may be a sign of other conditions and so should not be ignored) and lack of energy. Loss of muscle mass and weight gain can also contribute to fatigue and reduced energy.

Levels of hemoglobin may be corrected in part by a diet high in iron. Deep-green leafy vegetables can help, and red meat is also known to increase iron stores; but caution is needed if the man has heart disease or any other condition that requires him to avoid red meat. An iron supplement may be suggested by his primary care provider. Resistance training (yes, that again!) increases endurance and decreases fatigue.

WHAT COMES NEXT . . .

This has been a long and complex chapter. And the very nature of further treatments for prostate cancer can be depressing because it means that the cancer has come back or was advanced to begin with. Remember that many men live for years with advanced prostate cancer, and androgen deprivation therapy can help keep the cancer under control for a long time. In the next chapter you will read about participating in clinical trials or studies, which is often the route taken by men who have exhausted other forms of treatment and need something that is very new and still being tested.

· *10* ·

Will This Improve My Chances?

Enrolling in Clinical Trials

*W*hat does it mean to be in a clinical trial? How do you decide if this is right for your partner/spouse, and how do you deal with the uncertainty of not knowing if he is getting medication or a placebo (sugar pill)? The process of enrolling in a clinical trial, giving consent, and dealing with uncharted waters is discussed in this chapter.

Research is very important in the world of cancer; it's because of research that new drugs are found to help patients with cancer, and research has driven the improvements we have seen in cancer survivorship. We all know about the need for research into prostate cancer; the blue ribbon for prostate cancer research is almost as visible as the pink ribbon for breast cancer research. But really understanding what it means to participate in research, to be the subject of research, is another matter entirely.

The focus of this chapter is on research that tests one treatment against another or that tests a new drug to see if it is effective against cancer. This kind of research is called a clinical trial or study, and most advances in the treatment of cancer have come about because of this kind of research. There are other kinds of research too; asking a patient or caregiver to fill out a survey about their experiences as a cancer patient or interviewing a patient's family about the quality of the care provided in the hospital is also research; we learn from the participants how to do things better or differently.

WHAT IS A CLINICAL TRIAL?

Martin and Ina didn't expect to hear what the oncologist told them.

"Martin, we've exhausted all your options at this point. I'm sorry, but this happens sometimes. There are just some men, like you, whose cancer progresses no matter what we do in terms of treatment. Your cancer is now what we call "hormone resistant"—it continues to grow despite your being on hormone therapy. But there's a trial that you might benefit from, and I've asked Debra our research nurse to explain it to you. Is that okay? Can I bring her in?"

They sat there, unable to speak. It was as bad as the day four years ago when Martin learned he had prostate cancer. Dr. Gardiner took this as permission, and he picked up the phone on the desk, punched in a few numbers, and spoke quietly into the phone. A minute later there was a soft knock on the door, and a middle-aged woman in a white coat came into the room.

"Mr. Wilson. . . Mrs. Wilson . . . I'm Debra Worth, one of the research nurses here. Dr. Gardiner has asked me to talk to you about a clinical trial, a study of a new drug we're enrolling patients in. Are you interested in hearing about it?"

Neither Ina nor Martin knew what to say, so they just nodded in a distracted way. They both had so many questions about what Dr. Gardiner had said to them—Hormone resistant? The cancer was growing?—but the woman in the white coat was talking again, and they knew they should be listening.

A clinical trial tests whether a new treatment is safe and effective. The treatment may be a new chemotherapy drug, a new kind of radiation therapy, or a new way of giving medication or radiation. Before the researchers can begin to talk to potential participants, the researchers have to get approval for what they want to do from an institutional review board, which is often part of a university or may be a private company that reviews research. Members of the review board are usually doctors, researchers, and patient advocates, and they are independent of the researchers doing the trial. The review board ensures that the research is ethical and conducted according to the rules and laws that have been made to protect research participants.

This same review board will also monitor the trial to ensure that the researchers continue to do what they said they were going to do. If the trial is using a new medication or piece of equipment, the company that makes the product will also have a role to play in monitoring the trial and making sure that participants are receiving the appropriate tests and that everything is being documented correctly. The review board can also stop the study if the effects of the new drug or treatment are dangerous; they will also stop the study if the benefits from the new treatment are so great that other patients should receive it as soon as possible.

Clinical trials are divided into three kinds: phase 1, 2, and 3. In a phase 1 trial, participants (usually healthy volunteers) are given the new drug to see if it is safe and at what doses it can be given. Phase 1 trials often happen in the hospital or a special clinical trial unit where participants are given the drug and very closely monitored to see what side effects there are at various doses.

After the safety of the drug is shown from the phase 1 study, the medication moves into phase 2 testing. This is the stage where the effectiveness of the drug against the cancer is studied. Participation in phase 2 studies is usually offered to patients with advanced cancer who may benefit from the drug, but there is no guarantee that this will happen—the clinical trial is being done to see if the drug is effective.

The benefit to the patient/participant from phase 1 and 2 trials is very limited. The majority of those who take part in these trials see no improvements to their own health or disease progression, and it is estimated that only 5 percent experience any benefit at all and may in fact feel worse while on the experimental drug.[1]

Phase 3 clinical trials are the ones that you may be familiar with. In this type of study, the new drug is tested against existing drugs. There is always a control group (see the next section about randomization), and the participants with cancer are often newly diagnosed with cancer. This kind of trial is used to see if the new drug is more, less, or as effective as other drugs. It is often the only way that people with cancer can have access to new drugs, but there is no guarantee that the participant will get the new drug; he or she may get the older drug or even a placebo (sugar pill). This is due to the randomization process, which is very important for informing health-care providers that a new treatment is better than what we already have.

THE RANDOMIZATION PROCESS

In order to know whether one drug is better than another, it has to be tested in a randomized, controlled trial. There are two concepts here that are important to understand—randomization and control. Randomization refers to the process whereby participants are put into one (or more) groups purely by chance. While the actual process is complicated, randomization is done almost as if tossing a coin: the study participant has an equal chance of being in each group—the one that gets the new drug or the one that gets the current usual treatment. In cancer trials, the new or experimental drug is usually compared to an established drug; it would not be ethical to deny someone treatment by giving him a placebo.

The participant does not know what group he is in, and often his health-care providers and the researchers conducting the study also don't know. This is called "blinding" and is done to prevent any bias on the part of the health-care team who may be influenced if they know whether the patient is getting the experimental drug or not. All participants in the study get the same treatment (except for the drugs being tested) and monitoring while in the study.

———— ⟨⟩ ————

Jamie was a "can do" kind of man, and he didn't hesitate to agree to be part of a study investigating a new kind of chemotherapy for men with advanced cancer. He thought it was his best shot at beating the cancer, and he wanted to do that more than anything. He and Annie had met just last year on a Caribbean cruise for older singles, and he wanted to be around for a very long time with his new love.

He arrived early for all his appointments and was the life and soul of the treatment room—cracking jokes and making faces behind the nurses' backs to the great amusement of the other patients sitting in their chairs, hooked up to their IVs. The nurses loved him and always made a fuss over him. He acted as if what he was going through was no big deal, and he told them all that he was going to be just fine, that he would outlive even the youngest of the nurses.

He was devastated when his oncologist told him that his PSA was still going up—how could it? The doctor explained that the new medication didn't work for everyone, or perhaps he was not getting the experimental drug and that was why his cancer was continuing to grow. Jamie looked at him with confusion in his eyes.

"What do you mean, Doc? I'm in the study; I'm getting the new wonder drug, right?"

His doctor sighed deeply and sat down on a stool in front of Jamie.

"Jamie, remember when you discussed the study with the research nurse? Remember she told you that you would be randomized to either the active treatment group, the experimental treatment, or you might end up in the control group, the patients who get standard treatment? Well, we won't know which group you're in until the study is over, but you had an equal chance of not getting the experimental drug."

"What do you mean, Doc? What are you telling me? Please, Doc. . . . You met Annie. . . . I have to beat this, Doc; I have to!"

———— ⟨⟩ ————

The other important thing to know is that there is usually a control group that is compared to the experimental group (those getting the new treatment). The control group is made up of patients who get the standard treatment (or in rare cases, a placebo) and not the experimental drug. It is important to have this group as a comparison so that we know if the new drug is better, worse, or the same in treating the cancer. Some patients don't like the idea that they may be in this control group and think that this means they are not getting the "best" treatment. This is often a reason why patients refuse to participate in clinical trials—they think that they will be disadvantaged and don't want to take the risk that they are not getting the most effective treatment.[2] If we know that the new treatment is in fact better, this concern would be justified, but this kind of study is only done if we are not sure which treatment is better.

CONSENTING TO TAKE PART IN A TRIAL

Something else that is very important to understand about taking part in a clinical trial is the process of consenting to participation. We don't study anything about patients without their permission—and for a clinical trial, that means signing a form (or more than one form) indicating that the person has been told about the details of the trial, has understood what being part of the trial means, and is willing to take part in the trial. In other words, the person consents to participate and signs a consent form stating that.

The explanation of the trial can be long and fairly tedious—there are often many complicated concepts that have to be explained, and often the patient or his family don't fully understand what they are told. Part of the problem is that this explanation (or recruitment) is done at a time of high anxiety and confusion for the patient and his family. The man may have just learned that he has cancer, and now he has to make a decision to participate in a trial. Or perhaps he has just learned that the cancer is back, or that it is more serious than originally thought, and he has to think about taking part in a trial before the news has even sunk in. These are often times of helplessness, hopelessness, and distress, and so the reason for the trial, or what it might offer the patient, is confusing. This can lead the patient to consent for the wrong reasons.

Study participants who agree to take part in a study very quickly and don't take enough time to really consider what it means to be part of clinical research are more likely to not fully understand the implications of being part of a clinical trial. And they are also more likely to experience regret about their decision to participate.[3] This happens when decisions have to be made under life-threatening circumstances and the person really doesn't have the concentration or attention to understand the finer details of participation.[4]

———————❧———————

Dennis wasn't sure that he wanted to take part in the study that his urologist talked about—but his partner Alex didn't agree.

"Of course you want to do this, Den . . . it might make a difference to your chances, and it'll help other men like you."

"But what if I don't get the new drug? What if I get the sugar pill and I die anyway?"

Alex took a deep breath. Dennis was such a pessimist; he always expected the worst, and sometimes Alex thought that he created his own bad outcomes.

"Den . . . you heard the doctor. This may be your best chance! Dr. Bernard wouldn't have mentioned it if he didn't think it would benefit you. And you don't want to make an enemy of your doctor, do you? If he thinks you'll benefit, you should listen to him."

But Dennis wasn't convinced. The thought of being a guinea pig—and he didn't care what Alex or anyone else had to say, he would be a guinea pig—just made him uncomfortable. He was not going to do this, no matter how Alex tried to persuade him. He had made up his mind, and that was the end of that. He wanted to go home.

———————❧———————

Communication about the trial is a key part of the decision to participate or not. How the person introduces the topic and how he or she explains it is a key factor in whether someone agrees to take part in a clinical trial or not. The physician is usually the first person to mention to a patient that there is a clinical trial available; how effectively the physician communicates this information is very important in getting the patient to agree to hear more about the study or to be part of the study. One study found that it was the perceived friendliness of the physician and how easy it was for the patient to maintain a conversation with him or her that made the difference between agreeing or refusing to take part in a study.[5]

It is well accepted that when the treating physician recommends that a patient take part in a trial, this can be seen as coercive because the patient may think that if he doesn't agree, his care will be affected negatively. But studies suggest that this personal recommendation holds great weight for patients,[6] and messages from the physician that suggest that the physician, the patient, and the family are a team are highly influential in getting patients to agree to take part in a trial.[7]

A solution to this—and one demanded by some institutional review boards—is that the physician ask someone else, usually a research nurse who is not part of the patient's health-care team, to explain the study to the patient. In this way there is less chance that the patient will feel pressured or coerced to agree to participate. And the research nurse has been trained to explain the study in simple terms and to answer any questions that the patient and family have.

SHOULD YOUR PARTNER TAKE
PART IN A CLINICAL TRIAL?

People with cancer agree to be part of clinical trials for all sorts of reasons. They want to receive expert care and believe that being in a trial will allow them to receive that care. Some patients feel that they have no choice and that they have to take part in research to gain some personal benefit or because they think they have nothing to lose.[8] Others want to help by being part of the discovery of new knowledge about prostate cancer and its treatment. Some want to take part to please their health-care team or because their doctor or nurse recommended that they take part. Still others do it because they feel thankful to the hospital for providing them with care and want to show their gratitude by "paying back" the hospital.

But some men have no interest in agreeing to take part in a trial. One of the reasons for this is that they are not told about any trials by health-care providers. Some people are suspicious of research and feel like they would be experimented on. Other reasons include concern about the side effects of the experimental treatment, not trusting the researchers who are trying to recruit them into a trial, or not wanting to have repeated blood tests or other tests like scans. Some men find that having to travel to the hospital for additional appointments is burdensome and expensive if travel and parking are not paid for.[9] Other men don't want to place additional burden on their partner or family who would want or have to accompany them for study visits.[10] Whether the man agrees to participate or not, his care will not be affected in any way. This is important to know because some agree to participate because they are afraid that if they don't, their physician will be angry with them. This is one reason why it is important that someone other than the treating physician explain the study to the patient and answer all his (and your) questions.

The expectations of the participant for benefits from participation are important to consider. Clinical trials are conducted to increase knowledge and to test drugs and other treatments for all those who come after the participants in those trials. The studies are *not* designed to provide benefit to those who take part. This is a very altruistic goal and one that patients and families often don't understand. In a study that looked at the expectations of participants in a phase 1 clinical trial (remember that this kind of trial is done to assess the safety of the drug), participants expected that they would benefit from participation by seeing their tumor(s) get smaller and also that they would have more communication with their physician. This did not happen. They also expected that some of their symptoms would improve, but this also did not happen.[11]

Should You Influence His Decision?

Bernie had a family that he loved above everything else. His wife Rose and his children Tammy and Brian were the center of his life. They'd been at his side every step of the way through his cancer—one of them drove him to his appointments for the radiation therapy, and Rose always came with him to see the specialists. Tammy was getting married the following summer, and he wanted more than anything to walk her down the aisle. But he was tired, so tired, and after three years on the injections to stop his hormones, he was finished with treatment. He just wanted to be left alone with no more treatments and appointments and needles. But now they were offering him some kind of chemotherapy—and he had to agree to be part of a study to get the drug.

But his family would hear nothing about his quitting. His wife started to cry the first time he said he wasn't interested in chemotherapy; then she told the kids, and they started in on him. The worst was Tammy—she looked at him as if he'd slapped her, and then she walked off and didn't talk to him for a week. Brian and his wife Tiff flew in from Baltimore to try to persuade him—and the kicker was when Tiff told him that she was pregnant and that they wanted their child to know his or her grandfather. But he was tired—and he didn't want any more treatment—but how could he let them down?

———— ∞∞∞ ————

Pressure from family and friends may play a role in a man's decision to take part in a clinical trial even if he doesn't want to.[12] Communication may be at the root of these differences. Perhaps the family is desperate to keep the man with them under any circumstances, and they think that a clinical trial offers hope for that. They may not know all the details about the trial and think that he should be prepared to experience side effects in order to prolong his life. However, he may have other ideas, and it's important for you all to be on the same page about what he wants and what he doesn't want.

As hard as it may be to hear that he does not want to take part in a clinical study, remember that this is not a rejection of *you* but rather a reflection of how he feels about his cancer and his willingness to undergo further treatment. If he is tired and doesn't want to put himself through the rigors of more treatment and additional tests, then that is his decision, however difficult it is for you to accept. Keep in mind that clinical trials are often of little benefit to the participant himself but are rather about discovering new information that may help other men, so participation is a selfless act rather than one that benefits the participant.

WHAT QUESTIONS SHOULD YOU ASK ABOUT CLINICAL TRIALS?

Many people don't know what they should ask about taking part in clinical trials, so they keep quiet and accept what they are told and then make a decision based on partial information. The following are some questions suggested by the Johns Hopkins Medical Center and posted on their website:

- Who is funding the clinical trial?
- Why do researchers think the treatment may work?
- Will the treatment cause any pain? If so, for how long?
- What happens if the treatment is harmful?
- What medications, procedures, or treatments should be avoided during the clinical trial?
- Will clinical trial results be made available to participants and others?
- Can the treatment be continued after the clinical trial is over?
- What are the possible short- and long-term side effects?
- How do the risks and benefits of the investigative treatment compare with proven available treatments?
- What costs will be covered by the clinical trial (for travel or overnight stays, for example)?
- Will there be any remuneration?
- Will participation affect insurance or medical coverage?[13]

You may also want to know about how much time the various appointments will take and whether they can be scheduled at the same time as your partner's regular visits to the physician. He should be given the names and contact information of the research team and who to contact to find out more information. He should be provided with written information in the language of his choice, and this should be written at a level that you all can understand.

WHERE CAN YOU FIND MORE
INFORMATION ABOUT CLINICAL TRIALS?

There are other resources available to help you understand the processes involved in taking part in clinical trials as well as what trials are available and open to recruitment. ClinicalTrials.gov is a website of the National Institutes of Health that has reliable information for the public: http://www .clinicaltrials.gov. There is a similar website for Canadians at www.ontario .canadiancancertrials.ca.

WHAT COMES NEXT . . .

This chapter has explained the complicated issue of clinical trials. Many men with cancer and their partners will not have to even think about it; prostate cancer caught early has a high cure rate, and most men will not see their cancer progress to the point where experimental treatment is necessary. But there are also studies that compare one treatment to another—for example, can radiation therapy be given over three weeks instead of eight weeks—and men with early prostate cancer may be invited to participate in this kind of research. There are also studies of patient and partner satisfaction with the care provided, and you may be approached to take part in this kind of research that does not involve drugs. In the next chapter you will read about how to communicate effectively with your partner, your family members, and the health-care team. Communication is an important part of our everyday lives, so turn the page and get started.

· *11* ·

Let's Talk about It!

Communication

Communication is vitally important in all relationships, but especially when a couple's functioning is challenged by acute or chronic health problems. How do you start the conversation about a sensitive topic like sexual functioning? And how do you talk about what will happen if your spouse/partner is not doing well and needs help? Suggestions for these difficult conversations are provided in this chapter.

Communication is at the heart of everything we do—our relationships, our work, and receiving goods and services from everyone including the tax man and our hairdresser. Communication is at the very center of our primary relationships with our spouse/partner, and when illness happens, it becomes even more important to be able to communicate effectively. You'd think this would be easy—you love him and you've been together for ages—so why do you need to read a chapter on communication? Isn't this an automatic function of being human? What can you possibly learn about this at your stage of life? This chapter is about helping you communicate more effectively with your partner/spouse and also with health-care providers at this challenging time.

TALKING TO DOCTORS AND NURSES

Much of what you have read up to this point has been about providing you with information to help you understand what is happening with your partner's illness. But this is not the sum total of all that you could know; information often leads to questions, and I'm sure you've had reason and I hope opportunity to interact with the health-care providers who are treating your partner/spouse.

Communication in the medical setting requires both the health-care provider and the patient and partner to send messages to each other, and these messages are then interpreted and other messages are sent.[1] Each of the parties in this process is influenced by their own needs, values, beliefs, emotions, and skills. There are a multitude of external factors that also influence both the health-care provider and the patient. For the patient this might be irritation at having waited for an hour in the waiting room, anxiety about hearing test results, and worry about getting a parking ticket. For the physician, an external factor might be the knowledge that the clinic is running behind and the feeling of hunger in his/her stomach because he/she missed breakfast that morning. In addition, each of the parties has goals that they wish to achieve from the interaction; for the physician it may be getting as much information from the patient as possible in as short a time as possible. For the patient the goal may be to hear good news and to get out of the examination room as soon as possible. These goals are not the same. And the communication between patients and health-care providers takes place in an environment that has social, cultural, legal, and physical aspects that also play a role in what is said, what is heard, and how it is understood and interpreted. Taking into consideration all these factors, it is no wonder that communication is sometimes complicated and often not easy.

Everyone had told them that Dr. Black was the best in the business, but Rosemary couldn't figure out why. The man was like the Tasmanian Devil from the cartoons; he had rushed into the examination room where she and Gerald had been patiently waiting for thirty minutes, he hardly made eye contact, and then he rattled off a bunch of numbers, shook Gerald's hand, and left the room, banging the door closed as he left. They had looked at each other, and then Gerald laughed.

"Talk about bedside manner!"

But Rosemary didn't think it was funny. Gerald was on that active surveillance thing, and she was sure that he needed more information than they had just been given. Or had they been given anything? She surely didn't know any more than she had when they had been sitting waiting for the doctor to see Gerald.

Then a young woman who introduced herself as Dr. Black's assistant came in. She handed Gerald a piece of paper with numbers on it and a small card with the date and time of his next appointment.

"Any questions?" she asked as she backed toward the open door. "Okay then, see you next time!"

And she was gone.

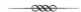

The interactions that you have with health-care providers are often rushed and on their terms, not yours. Surgeons and oncologists run very busy clinics, and often they only allot ten minutes (or even less) to each patient. This doesn't leave much time for talking or having your questions answered. There are some ways to get the attention you need, and this section of the chapter is going to focus on that; how to communicate effectively with busy health-care providers is a skill and an art, and there is probably very little in your past that has prepared you for it.

Medical Vocabulary

In order to be able to communicate effectively with health-care providers, you're going to have to learn some of the words and phrases that are commonly used. Yes, these health-care providers should be the ones to explain them to you, but that won't necessarily happen. A good medical dictionary will be a great help in this regard. Most public libraries have them in the reference section, and you can also find them online (see the "Resources" section at the end of this chapter). For example, sometimes a doctor will say that a test is "negative," and by that he/she means that the result was normal and there is nothing wrong. But most people interpret a "negative" result as meaning that there is something wrong. The same applies to the word "positive" when it applies to a test; a positive result in this case may mean that there is something wrong!

You need to have a basic working knowledge of the terms used most commonly in the world of prostate cancer. Hopefully if you have read all the chapters in this book you will be familiar with the most common terms like *biopsy, radical prostatectomy*, and so forth. Think of it as being like visiting a foreign country; you don't need to be an expert in the language of that country, but it helps if you recognize the word for ladies' restroom.

Here are some resources for you that may help with learning this new language:

http://www.nlm.nih.gov/medlineplus/mplusdictionary.html
    From the NIH and the National Library of Medicine
http://www.medterms.com/script/main/hp.asp
    A trustworthy site associated with *Webster's Medical Dictionary*

http://medical-dictionary.thefreedictionary.com/
> Another trustworthy source associated with a well-known medical dictionary for health-care providers.

Demanding Clear Communication

When Michael was diagnosed three months earlier, he'd heard the results on the phone. Dr. Brooks the urologist had called him during dinner on Tuesday night to say that his biopsy was positive and that he'd like to see Michael and his wife on Friday afternoon at 5:30. Michael's wife, Diana, who had worked as a nurse for thirty-five years thought that was a little strange. An appointment at 5:30 on a Friday afternoon meant that dinner with the grandchildren would have to be canceled; but the next minute the shock of what the doctor had told Michael set in, and she had to sit down for a bit.

Prostate cancer! They didn't talk about it much over the few days before Friday was upon them. Michael didn't like to talk about health stuff, so in the meantime, Diana had read what she could find in the local library. By Friday she had a pretty good idea about what they were dealing with, and she had made a list of questions for the doctor. She didn't tell Michael about the questions—he got irritated when she used her nursing background around him—but she knew that he would just sit and listen and not ask any questions. He was really passive when it came to his health, and she knew that this was serious and that someone had to stand up and be counted this time.

And as she predicted, Michael just sat there as the doctor talked. But she had to admit that Dr. Brooks knew his stuff. He was patient and stopped to ask if they had any questions as he explained about the PSA and the Gleason score. He didn't seem at all rushed, and he even seemed pleased when she pulled out her list of questions.

"Ah, a test for me! I like that! So go ahead, please. Fire away!"
She liked this Dr. Brooks. She liked him a lot.

Some health-care providers take great pains to communicate clearly to patients and family members, and they do a good job. Some physicians keep the last appointment of the day for newly diagnosed patients so that they can take as much time as needed to explain the diagnosis and treatment options. Others set aside time each week to see patients who are having a difficult time or whose cancer has come back, as they recognize that these patients may need extra time and explanations. But other physicians just can't be bothered (or just act like that) or think that patients should be able to understand them in a quick consultation, and so they don't make special arrangements for the patient. This is not an excuse, but physicians are a product of their training and education, and they are a product of where they originated from and the cultural norms they grew up in. Some societies are more hierarchical than others, and some physicians may have been trained to believe and act as if they are the ones in charge and that patients and other health-care providers (like nurses) have to obey them. A study from Spain found that specialists tend to act in a managerial style and don't ask about their patients' emotions or expectations. These doctors showed a very limited range of communicative skills and paid little attention to the needs of their patients.[2]

This is where you come in: You have to be the primary advocate for your spouse or partner. As mentioned over and over in the previous pages, you must go with him to all appointments to act as a second set of ears, a recorder of verbal discussions, and the prompter of new questions. Your role is vital—because most people under duress (a diagnosis of cancer is a situation of duress) forget to ask questions and have a hard time remembering to speak for themselves or to report new symptoms to the health-care provider. You don't have to speak for your partner all the time—but you have his best interests at heart and so can act as a backup coach or secretary.

Seeking Clarification

It may be easier for you to ask for clarification if either of you doesn't understand something because you have just enough distance from the physical sensations to be able to speak up. It may be that you see things differently from your partner/spouse; perhaps you don't hold the same ideas about the doctor as the boss of the situation and so you are willing to take the risk of interrupting the flow of information when you need clarification of a word or statement. Your mate may be too tense or too anxious to keep his thoughts in order, or he may be intimidated by the seriousness of the situation and not want to ask because he is afraid to hear the answer.

One way of seeking clarification is paraphrasing what you have just heard. So saying something like, "What I just heard you say is . . . ," allows the physician to think about what you understood by his or her words. If there was a misunderstanding or lack of clarity, this can then be corrected. You can also ask for more details—"Can you explain that further?"—or seek more information with a phrase like, "What happens if . . . ?"

How to Ask Questions

In this foreign world (to you) of cancer, the doctors and nurses are the experts, and sometimes it can feel intimidating to ask questions. You may not want to seem as if you are questioning the doctor's authority or expertise, and there are some physicians who are really good at making you feel inferior. Being able to advocate for your partner and yourself requires a combination of assertiveness and diplomacy.

There are a number of ways to ask questions. One study[3] showed that the questions asked in an interaction with a medical specialist were of two kinds. The first is for the patient to be direct and ask his question. The second is to raise the general topic in conversation so that either of you may be able to indirectly get the information you need. The study found that 41 percent of patients observed asked a direct question (mostly about diagnostic tests) and 18 percent asked their question indirectly. When the number of questions in the interaction was counted, it was observed that the medical specialist asked nine questions (about physical symptoms), the patient asked four questions, and the companion managed to ask just one question.

Remember that the doctor works for *you*. You have chosen him or her to provide your partner/spouse with a service, and the doctor has a contract with you and your spouse to provide good service. You can always go somewhere else for that service (depending of course on where you live or the limits imposed by your health-care insurance). But because a doctor deals with health and illness, and in this case a serious illness, we often forget which way the power flows and get intimidated by the doctor's qualifications or importance. Thinking about this may help you to be more assertive and aware of where the power really lies.

But you can't be rude, as this often puts people's backs up. Be diplomatic and choose your words carefully. Ask your questions when there is a gap in the conversation, not when the doctor is in midsentence. But sometimes it needs to be broken. Lots of physicians have learned to avoid questions by not leaving the patient the time to get a question into the conversation. Sometimes you need to be a little aggressive to be heard. If the answer doesn't provide you with the information you need or asked for, ask again. "Please tell me why . . . ?" or "Can you please repeat that?" are respectful and nonaggressive phrases that invite further explanation and don't put the health-care provider on the defensive.

It is always a good idea to write down all your questions before the appointment and keep them in order of priority. Tell the doctor at the start of the appointment that you have some questions that you would like to ask before the appointment is over. Some physicians have a policy of not allowing the patient's spouse/partner to be in the room during a physical examination. This may result in your being ushered out before you get a chance to ask your questions, or you may not be invited into the room at all. In this case it may be helpful to make another appointment just to ask the questions. Explain this to the receptionist when you call to book an appointment, and you may be given the last appointment of the day so that there is enough time.

You are often aware that the waiting room you just sat in was full of other patients waiting to be seen; be mindful that the physician knows this too and may be feeling pressured to keep moving in order to see all his patients in a limited time. The full waiting room may be a result of poor planning on his part, but it could also be because he/she saw an emergency case that interrupted the flow of patients. If you have a lot of questions, tell the doctor this at the beginning of the appointment and say that you would be willing to come back at another time, but you don't want to wait too long. However, if your questions are urgent or about matters that you think are urgent, you have a right to have them answered, even at the risk of making others wait longer.

Time (or the lack of it) is a major issue in health care. There is just not enough time in our lives, it seems, and there are many reasons why this is not dealt with effectively by health care providers.[4] Lack of time with the physician causes a great deal of patient dissatisfaction, an increase in malpractice claims, and physician dissatisfaction too. When physicians feel short on time, they show signs of stress and annoyance (which the patient can see or feel), and they hurry in and out of rooms, ask their questions in a rushed way, hurry through any physical examination, and frequently interrupt the patient when he is talking.

TALKING TO EACH OTHER

So, you've been with this same man for ten or twenty or even fifty years and you each know how the other thinks, right? Perhaps at times you even say the exact same thing at the exact same time and you both laugh at how well you know each other. But when illness occurs, those automatic and familiar ways of communicating often don't work any longer or as effectively. Times of crisis require *great* communication, not just good communication, and it requires the use of words rather than looks or telepathy.

"Honey, what is it? You've been so quiet lately. Is it me? Have I done something wrong?"

"For goodness' sake, it's nothing. Why do you always think that it's something? Can't a man just be quiet?"

"But honey, you're not acting like it's nothing. You're withdrawn. You're not talking to me. I know, it's because I bought those shoes."

"It's not the damn shoes! It's nothing! Can't you just leave it alone?"

"Oh my goodness . . . it's the cancer, isn't it? You've found out something about the cancer and you don't want to tell me because I'll get upset! Well, I'm upset already so you might as well just spit it out!"

And then the sound of the door slamming . . .

Studies have shown that the partners of men with prostate cancer are often more distressed than the man himself. Cancer changes everything—how confident we are in the future, our notions of certainty in the world—and prostate cancer has the added stressor of affecting masculinity and the sex life of the couple. Death and sex are two difficult topics to talk about—and prostate cancer brings both to the forefront. We know that many couples actively try to avoid talking about death and sex—and so often they don't talk about prostate cancer either.[5] This is sometimes dependent on the stage of the disease process—there is more talk in the early stages and less after treatment. It is thought that this may have something to do with many men's desire to get back to life as usual and their reluctance to talk about their feelings.[6]

Over time, our communication patterns become entrenched, and not always in a good way. One of you may be the "talker," and the other the "silent partner." In times of stress, the "talker" may need to hear what the other person is thinking or feeling; he or she may need the "silent" one to be more communicative and sharing. But the "silent partner" may find solace in keeping quiet and trying to figure out things for him- or herself. So the "talker" talks more and demands more, and the "silent partner" withdraws more and more. These are old patterns that are not effective in new and difficult situations.

The meaning of the illness can have a significant impact on the communication of the couple. If the man treats the disease as a minor inconvenience that will be dealt with quickly and effectively with surgery but his partner interprets the diagnosis as a threat to his life that therefore puts her at risk of becoming a widow, you can see how they would think about it quite differently and of course talk (or avoid talking) about it differently too. Wanting to talk, and in turn avoiding talking, can reduce relationship closeness and increase distress.[7] It is at times of stress and crisis that partners need to be connected to each other, what we call relationship intimacy, but communication problems can drive the couple apart.

Here are some tips for improving communication:

- *Make time to talk.* Whatever needs to be said is important, so treat the conversation like you would a meeting or appointment. Sit down together with no distractions: cell phones off, house telephone going to the answering machine, and TV and radio off—not just on mute. Sit down; you'd be surprised at how standing to talk makes the conversation feel intimidating to some.
- *Talk in "I" statements.* You've probably heard this a thousand times—but we often talk about what the other person has done or assume what he is thinking and we are completely wrong. When you start a sentence with, "You make me feel . . . ," the other person feels picked on and will naturally get defensive. A much better way of saying something is, "I feel so alone when you keep quiet and don't tell me what you're thinking." This puts the emotion (and blame) on yourself and allows the other person some wriggle room instead of feeling like he's in a corner of the boxing ring and you're in front of him, swinging away.
- *Name the problem.* Before you start talking, figure out what exactly you want to talk about. That might sound a little silly, but we often avoid these conversations, and so when we eventually have them, we can't really remember what the major issue is. We instead present a smorgasbord of issues to our partner, and this feels overwhelming and even threatening. Is the issue that you are worried about him because you don't know what he is thinking? Or are you mad at him because he opted to just watch his cancer instead of treating it aggressively?
- *Listen.* It sounds simple, and I bet you thought you were doing that all along. But we often don't really listen to what our partner is telling us, and we often don't pay attention to his body language and nonverbal behavior. After you've said what you want to talk about or what is bothering you, make a conscious effort to stop talking. Silence can be uncomfortable for many people, and if one person just keeps quiet, the other one will often jump in and say something to break the silence. But when he starts to talk, don't jump in. Just stay silent and let him talk. Men in our society have been socialized to take control of conversations—if you just let him talk, he will tell you what you need to know, most of the time.
- *Be flexible in your response.* You may not get exactly what you want from the conversation—he may be determined to avoid surgery, and if you give him a chance, he'll tell you why. It may not be what you want to hear, but you'll be hearing it from him, and that was the point of having the conversation in the first place.
- *Avoid nitpicking.* There is a big difference between having a fight or argument and slowly and consistently picking away at minor issues

without seeking resolution. Picking on multiple, small issues instead of addressing one or two (or even more) big issues is not productive. It may cause him to withdraw even further and leave you feeling frustrated and bitter.

• *Control your emotions.* This is a difficult one because you may be very upset and worried and frustrated, and when you start to talk, you may cry or shout or hyperventilate. Remember that men, particularly those of a certain age, have been taught how to respond to others' emotions by the messages they received growing up as children. So their tendency is to "suck it up" and not show their emotions, so they have a hard time dealing with emotion in others. It makes them feel helpless and they don't know what to do, so they often withdraw, which is exactly what you don't need.

HOW TO HAVE DIFFICULT CONVERSATIONS

There are specific concerns related to prostate cancer that necessitate difficult conversations. Talking about sex is not easy for most couples, and many couples have never had an open and honest conversation about something they have been doing for years. I often tell my patients that even though we are humans with pretty advanced capacity for verbal communication, when it comes to sex we are like whales and dolphins—we communicate in grunts and squeaks. We know from experience what the moans and sighs mean and so instead of saying "that feels really good" or "could you please lighten your touch," we change the sounds we make, and hopefully our partner gets it right. But when there are challenges, we discover that the grunts and squeaks are not helpful, and then we don't have the words.

As I wrote in my book *Woman Cancer Sex*,[8] talking about sensitive matters often requires not only honesty but also a balance between praise and criticism:

> There are different ways of saying things and how you say something can really influence how the message is received. "You make me crazy with your demands for sex" has a very different tone from "I don't want sex as often as you seem to." Sometimes in talking about sex we have to say things that may seem hurtful or may appear to our partner as a criticism. Balancing the positive and the negative is a delicate balance but if done carefully, can protect feelings and reduce the risk of causing hurt.

As you have read in previous chapters, the sexual side effects of the various treatments for prostate cancer are significant, and if the couple doesn't talk about what has changed and how this has affected both of them, then alternatives will not be found and a sexless relationship may be the result. This may be okay for some couples, but it is often the beginning of a gradual drifting apart. In a study of the partners of men with prostate cancer,[9] more than half of participants reported that they were unable to negotiate a new way of being sexual when penetrative intercourse was no longer possible. The other half of participants described finding ways to be sexual by falling back on activities that were secondary to "real sex" like masturbation, oral sex, and kissing and hugging. The challenges to this negotiation were identified as communication, sexual problems that were present before the diagnosis of cancer, and the partner seeing the man with cancer as a sick person who was no longer a sexual person. Those couples who were able to negotiate a satisfying sexual relationship said that while it was not easy to talk about, being open about their needs and desires was rewarding and brought about positive changes to not only the sexual relationship but the relationship generally.

Marlene didn't know where to turn or who to talk to. Things had been so different between her and Travis since his surgery. And he wouldn't talk about it no matter how hard she tried. He had never been one to talk about his feelings, but they had had a loving relationship throughout their marriage—and now things were very different.

The next time he went to his support group, she went too. She had gone with him to these meetings after they first found out about the cancer, but then she got busy with Christmas and stopped going. And after his surgery was over, there didn't seem to be much point. But she'd seen the e-mail about the next meeting, and the topic that the guest speaker was talking about was "intimacy." She realized that this was what was missing in their relationship. Travis hadn't touched her for . . . how long had it been? Certainly more than a few weeks, and as she thought about it, she realized that it had been closer to three months!

The hospital boardroom where the support group meetings were held was full to capacity. Everyone was interested in this topic it seemed! Travis looked most uncomfortable as the speaker started talking—but for Marlene it seemed as if the speaker was speaking directly to her! She described their situation perfectly—the withdrawal, the lack of touch, the silences, the undressing in the bathroom. . . . And the speaker explained why it was happening and what could be done to change the situation. For the first time in ages, Marlene felt like she had something to work with. She could hardly wait to get Travis in the car to start talking.

For men, the ability to function sexually is closely linked to their feelings of being a man. Changes in sexual functioning impact how they see themselves, and this can be very difficult to talk about because men are usually socialized to not discuss their feelings or show emotion, as this further diminishes their masculinity. Women often recognize this, perhaps after an attempt to talk about things, and don't raise the topic again because they see the hurt it causes. Women tend to report that they are more concerned about the effect of sexual difficulties on their partner than on themselves, and men often assume that if the woman doesn't complain, then she is not affected by the changes in their sex life.[10]

So how do you talk about something that is so emotionally loaded? You use the same strategies listed earlier in this chapter, but this may not be enough. Many couples find that they need professional help to talk about something as sensitive as sex. A social worker, psychologist, or counselor may be helpful to get you started talking in a meaningful way. A family or marital therapist may be an even better choice because they are trained in couple dynamics as well as communication. And perhaps a certified sex therapist or counselor may be the best bet of all because these professionals are also experts in human sexuality and will be able to help you communicate and provide suggestions to help you overcome sexual difficulties. You can find a certified sex therapist or counselor in your area by going to the website of the American Association of Sex Educators, Counselors and Therapists at www .AASECT.org. You can also start by writing a letter to your partner, expressing your feelings. This is a good way to formulate what you want to say, but it also gives you time to reflect on what you are thinking and feeling. You can give your partner the letter to read, you can read it to him, or you can just use the letter writing as a process to support what you want to communicate to him. By letting him read the letter, it also allows him time to think about what he will say in response.

Another difficult conversation to have is one about death, and unfortunately for some couples, this is a conversation that must be had when treatment fails and the cancer progresses despite everything that is tried. No one wants to have this conversation, but there are important matters to discuss—what, if any, intervention does he want if he stops breathing or his heart stops beating? We should all discuss our thoughts about this before a crisis occurs, and one way of doing this is to create a living will or advanced health-care directive that describes what if any measures should be taken (for example, CPR or antibiotics in case of infection) if and when we cannot speak for ourselves. This document goes hand in hand with a durable power of attorney for health care that names someone (often the partner) as the person who knows and will speak for the wishes of the patient if he cannot talk for himself. In order to fulfill the requirements of this proxy statement, you need to know what he would want if he were not able to talk for himself and decisions about treatment have to be made.

Caring Connections, a program of the National Hospice and Palliative Care Organization (NHPCO), is a national consumer and community engagement initiative to improve care at the end of life. This organization (www.caringinfo.org) provides free resources and information to help people make decisions about end-of-life care and services. The website has a number of useful resources including suggestions for hospice care in your area as well as Advanced Health Care Directives that are legal in different states.

It can be very difficult for men to talk about impending death, in part because they may see this as letting you down and not being there to take care of you as they have been socialized to do and have done lovingly for many years. If he won't talk about it, respect his wishes, but take the opportunity to tell him how you feel and how much you will miss him. Sometimes people who are dying hang on to life even when health-care providers tell you that they are going to die very soon. He may need permission to let go and leave you, and even though this may be the hardest thing you have ever had to do, you may need to tell him that it's okay to let go, that you will miss him terribly and love him, but that you will be okay without him—because eventually you will be okay.

WHAT COMES NEXT . . .

In the next chapter you will read about support groups, something that many couples engage in along their journey with prostate cancer. Support groups can serve different functions for different people, and this chapter will help you to understand the pros and cons of participating in these groups, which have become a major part of the cancer experience for many.

· *12* ·

One of the Guys

Joining a Support Group

.*M*any men are advised to attend a support group for prostate cancer patients/survivors. Is this right for your partner/spouse? And how about you? What do you hope to get out of attending a support group? How do you know what support group is right for either of you? This chapter will present the pros and cons of attending a support group and provide you with strategies to assess the quality and content of these groups.

Many men are advised to find a support group when they are diagnosed with prostate cancer. At times of heightened anxiety and uncertainty, most of us look for support from others, and if that support is provided by those who have "been there and done that," it is perhaps of even greater value than the support of family and friends who have not walked the same path. This chapter will describe the benefits of attending a support group for both of you, even though most of the research on this topic largely ignores the benefits for spouses/partners.

WHY GO TO A SUPPORT GROUP?

Roberto was not sure that this was the right thing for him, but his wife Luiza insisted that they go to the support group. She worked with a woman named Connie, and this woman's husband had gone and they just loved it.

"Connie says that they've met such nice people, people just like us. And she says that they've learned a lot. Connie's husband was going to get the surgery, but then he went to the meeting and he did something else."

Roberto was getting tired of "Connie said" and "Connie's husband," but once Luiza got an idea in her head, he knew he just needed to do what she wanted. Otherwise she would go on and on, and eventually he would do what she wanted just to stop the talking and talking.

So they went to the meeting, and he was surprised to see many men like him: younger (he was only fifty-six!) and Hispanic, and they all looked pretty good. It was a little awkward at first, but then they started joking around about how they were all dragged there by their wives and it got better. It didn't even feel like it was a meeting at first—they just stood around talking—but then a lady got up and said she was a social worker from the hospital, and they all stopped talking. And then he realized that they were all the same, all the men in that room. They all had cancer, and this was no laughing matter.

A primary role of support groups for men with prostate cancer has been the provision of education about the various treatment options available to them. Topics typically discussed at meetings include different kinds of treatment, coping with the quality-of-life challenges such as erectile problems and incontinence, new drugs available, complimentary therapies, the latest advances in diagnosis and treatment, and so forth. Benefits of attending a support group are thought to be increased social support, decreased social isolation, increased personal empowerment, increased self-esteem, and a decrease in negative mood.

But being part of a support group can be a double-edged sword. For men who go to a support group *before* they make a treatment decision, the information they receive can be very helpful in weighing the various options. For men who first go to a support group meeting *after* their treatment and realize that perhaps they had other options that they were not informed about, this knowledge can be distressing. Men who attended support groups said that since attending, they were more assertive about their own health and were less judgmental about others.[1]

Cancer support groups in general are said to provide a sense of community that is unique and different from the usual community that includes others without cancer. Being in a support group also provides a sense of being accepted and not feeling different, because everyone in the group has been directly affected by cancer. And of course there is the provision of information, not only about cancer but also about how to be a cancer patient or survivor—how to act and advocate for oneself, how to access the best care, and how to challenge the medical establishment when necessary.[2]

Another important aspect of attending a support group is the opportunity to learn how to be an astute health-care consumer. Many older men (and women) have not been socialized to question or confront health-care providers. From the preceding chapters, you have learned that there is often no right or wrong way to treat prostate cancer and that men are expected to learn about their choices and then make a choice about treatment. Support groups provide the opportunity for men to learn to question health-care providers and advocate for themselves, when their natural tendency may be to go with the attitude that "the doctor knows what's best for me."[3]

Some support groups use humor as an effective mechanism to balance and diffuse emotional and sensitive situations or topics. A recent study suggests that humor is effective for putting men at ease when they join a support group and don't yet know the norms and conventions of the group. Jokes were used to signal the boundary for talking about a sensitive topic like sexuality and also when the emotions among members became an issue. Humor was also used to normalize usually embarrassing experiences such as incontinence. Not all support group members appreciate the use of humor to deflect emotion, and there are times when something intended to be funny can be offensive to someone.[4] How partners/spouses interpret the humor was not highlighted in this study, but this is something that can cause trouble for couples. While men may find that joking about a sensitive topic like sexual functioning is helpful to lighten the mood and avoid embarrassment, their partner may feel that this is not appropriate.

But men with cancer tend to underutilize support groups; in one study it was found that only 13 percent of men attended at least one support group meeting (compared to 33 percent of women).[5] This may result from men being socialized to deal with their own problems without asking for help or support. Some men may not be aware of the existence of support groups, particularly if their health-care providers do not tell them about the support groups that are active in their area. Many physicians don't refer their patients to a support group—either because they don't know what's available or because they're concerned that what the patient might learn from the support group might change their treatment choice.[6]

Some people like to hear about others' experiences—they feel that they can learn more about what to expect in their own journey and how to cope with the various challenges inherent in the process before and after their treatment for prostate cancer. Both you and your partner/spouse may find role models within the support group whose experience closely mirrors your own, and you can learn from their successes and even their failures. Knowing that there are others who have been through a similar experience can reduce your sense of isolation and provide you with hope for the future. But there is a potential downside too—hearing about others who have not done well or who continue to experience bothersome side effects can be negative for both of you and may be a source of distress or anxiety.

Support groups are not for everyone, but many men say that they have benefited from attending—or else their partners have benefited, which is also important. Some people find support in other places—their church, for example—and there is still resistance among some men toward sharing personal details with strangers, or having their partner talk about the details of their life.

PARTNERS AND SUPPORT GROUPS

Is it necessary for you to go with your partner to a support group for men with prostate cancer? The answer to that question is that it depends both on the structure of the group and your expectations of the group. In the limited research that has been done on partners' participation in prostate cancer support groups,[7] the partners have exclusively been women, so we don't know if this applies to homosexual partners of men with prostate cancer.

Most women accompany their partner to a support group on the advice of a health-care provider, family member, or friend—or because it's the only way that their reluctant partner will attend a meeting himself. Women say that they go to learn about the disease and its management and to help their spouses/partners learn about their treatment choices. But women also go to learn from others' experiences about how to support their partner/spouse and also to gain support from other women. Some women initially go alone if their partner/spouse refuses to attend and hope that eventually he will start going too. This doesn't always happen, but if the woman's needs for support and information are being met, she may continue to attend by herself because of the benefits she receives from participation.

By attending support groups, you can hear the same information as your partner and become more knowledgeable about the disease and what to expect without having to take an active part in discussions. What you hear can then form the basis of conversations between the two of you, and you will have an opportunity to voice your concerns or provide support to him because you have this common knowledge. Hearing the stories of other couples can provide hope and reassurance that you too will get through the experience—but of course there is a downside when other couples don't fare that well. Many women find that they create new friendships with other women at these groups—an unplanned but pleasant by-product for many. These friendships form an extended support network comprised of others who have "been there and done that," and this is different from other friends who do not share the cancer experience.

Jerry had been the one who insisted that his wife Maura go with him to the support group meetings. That was over fifteen years ago, and now the monthly meetings were a regular part of their social life. Jerry's treatment was long over, but they had made so many friends in the group over the years, and most of those couples were still attending the meetings. Now Maura was the editor of the group newsletter, and Jerry was serving his second term as president. It was interesting to meet the new people who were often so scared that their faces were pinched and they didn't say much. Maura liked to see how they loosened up over the months and became part of the group. She could also tell which of the couples would go to just one or two meetings and then never come back. She knew that everyone had a right to do what was good for them—but the group had been such an important part of their life that she felt almost rejected when a couple didn't keep coming to the meetings, month after month, like Jerry and her. Oh well, such is life.

While most women initially take a "backseat" to the activities of the group, over time many begin to play specific roles—from welcoming new members, helping to make other women feel comfortable, serving refreshments, and organizing social activities like Christmas parties, to becoming part of the formal structure of the group and being involved in executive committees or the support group newsletter. If the support group is structured in a way that has the women meeting separately for part of the time, this is also an opportunity for you to share the fears and concerns that perhaps you don't want your partner/spouse to know about. It's not that you're hiding things from him, but sometimes not sharing your fears is safer for both of you—as long as you have somewhere to talk about these fears and also to learn how best to deal with them.

WHAT KIND OF SUPPORT GROUPS ARE THERE?

Since the 1990s, a number of support groups have started across North America and around the world. Support groups are basically of two kinds: there are those that are led by some sort of professional facilitator, perhaps a nurse or social worker, and those that are led by laypeople, for example a man who has had prostate cancer. Many support groups for men with prostate cancer strongly mirror businesses—they tend to have an executive committee with various roles (secretary, newsletter editor, etc.) and as such form a framework similar to the work that older men did before retirement.

Some prostate cancer support groups encourage spouses/partners to attend meetings for either the entire meeting or part of the meeting. It is not uncommon for the support group to be in two parts—an educational session where a health-care provider or other professional presents some kind of education about an aspect of prostate cancer and then a second part that is more supportive. It is often for this part that the men have a separate session from the partners/spouses (often assumed to be the female partners/wives). This of course presumes that only heterosexual men attend these support groups!

In the United States there are two major networks of prostate cancer support groups: Us TOO and Man to Man (which is part of the American Cancer Society). Us TOO also has a support network for the partners of men with prostate cancer: Us TOO Partners. Us TOO is a grassroots self-help organization that is run by prostate cancer survivors, and some larger cities may have two or more support groups under their umbrella. Their website (www .ustoo.com) has a lot of information about support groups in your area as well as information about prostate cancer, clinical trials, and other resources.

The Man to Man support groups can be found on the American Cancer Society website (http://www.cancer.org/Treatment/SupportProgramsServices/ MantoMan/index). This website is a little more difficult to navigate because the American Cancer Society is not strictly prostate cancer focused, but you can access the Man to Man newsletters, which offer good information, from this site.

Phoenix 5 is another network of prostate cancer support groups (http:// www.phoenix5.org/supportgroups.html). Out with Cancer (http://www .outwithcancer.com) is an organization for gays, lesbians, and bisexual survivors with cancer. While not a formal support group, information about resources specific to this population can be accessed on the website once you have registered as a member.

CancerCare is another organization that provides support for people with all kinds of cancer, and they offer a number of different support groups (online, in person, and by telephone) for men with prostate cancer (http:// www.cancercare.org/support_groups). The Cancer Hope Network (http:// www.cancerhopenetwork.org) is another not-for-profit organization that matches cancer patients and their families with trained volunteers; however it is not specific to prostate cancer.

ONLINE SUPPORT GROUPS

Online support groups have grown in both number and popularity. There are many reasons for this—the ease and convenience of twenty-four-hour access 365 days a year, no need for travel to a meeting, being able to seek support or information from the privacy of one's home at a time that is most convenient, the ability to remain anonymous without fear of stigma or judgment, and the potential to "lurk" without feeling that you have to participate. There are also potential downsides to this anonymity—concerns have been raised about privacy issues, the potential for spam and hoaxes, aggression and hostility, and the quality and validity of the information provided by peers.[8]

Cancer patients who use online support groups are also more likely to be white, highly educated, and with high household income.[9] Men with prostate cancer tend to use online support groups to find information related to specific problems or questions. Their interest seems to lie in accessing information rather than emotional support, and they see the Internet as a relatively private space where they feel comfortable sharing personal information.[10] In a study from Germany, men who accessed a support website for prostate cancer mostly sought information about treatment.[11] Sixty-six percent of questions were about treatment recommendations, but 46 percent of the questions were requests for emotional support. The answers from other participants reflected less emotional support (37 percent of responses) but personal experiences were shared by 28 percent.

Increasingly there are web-based support groups that provide similar support in terms of information. The Association of Cancer Online Resources (ACOR) (www.ACOR.org) was started to provide online support and education to people affected by different kinds of cancer. The organization has access to 159 mailing lists and through these encourages cancer survivors and their caregivers to communicate with each other on a variety of topics related to the specific cancer of interest.

The "New" Prostate Cancer Info Link (http://prostatecancerinfolink .net) is a website that was started by a Florida urologist that has multiple discussion forums and a "social network" that includes a section for wives and partners. Membership is required to participate in these discussion forums, but it is easy to register and become a member.

What about the use of online support groups by the partners/spouses of men with prostate cancer? Female relatives and friends of men with prostate cancer are active in online support groups for men, and they post messages on these websites more frequently and in greater detail and length than the men with prostate cancer themselves. The nature of the communication also reflects a general agreement with "typical" female communication style—warm greetings, discussion of personal feelings, and more efforts to support others. However, women on these "male" websites tend to use more male language and show restraint in their use of emotive language as compared to women in a breast cancer online support forum.[12]

Women who participate in support groups specifically for cancer caregivers seem to allow themselves to be more traditionally "female" in their postings. In these kinds of support groups, women tend to post personal messages reflecting their struggles with the caregiving role, their need for and appreciation of hope, and their experiences of the "emotional roller coaster" of the cancer experience. These support groups by virtue of their relative anonymity allow women to vent their feelings and talk about their sadness, frustration with their spouse or the system, and their anger at the cancer itself.[13] Women may find that their need for support increases if and when their spouse/partner gets sicker. If the demands on them for caregiving increase, there is a risk that they may become more isolated and so turn to online support groups for help in trying times.[14]

Vincent was still reeling from the shock of being diagnosed with prostate cancer; he was HIV positive and had been for more than twenty years, and he really thought that this was going to be what killed him. So a diagnosis of cancer on top of the HIV was just too much. His partner of thirty years, Les, was shocked too. But his response to the diagnosis was to go into "fact finding" mode, and he started searching for information on the Internet and in the medical library. Vincent didn't want to know anything. He went into a deep denial about what was happening and wouldn't talk about it or even go back to see the urologist. And he forbade Les to talk about it to anyone—not their friends or the few family members that they were in contact with. He made Les swear that he would not talk about it at work or at the gym or anywhere. This had to be a secret.

One night at 3 a.m. when Les was searching for more information on the Internet, he found a reference to an online support group. And just like that he clicked on the link and found this website where there was a live chat room as well as other pages with all sorts of information. He quickly registered and within minutes was reading the comments from other partners of men with prostate cancer. And there were five people in the live chat room. They all seemed to be women—but with a name like Les, they might not know he was a man—so he quickly typed a greeting before he lost his nerve.

So what might you gain from participating in online support groups? First there is the opportunity to learn about prostate cancer from those who are "walking the walk and talking the talk." This information should be read and interpreted critically—everyone has a different experience based on their own personality, life experience, level of knowledge, values, and attitudes. You can be a "lurker" and not post anything yourself and instead read and learn from others' postings. If you want to be more active, you can ask others how they have dealt with the concerns that you are experiencing. You can seek spiritual support if that is part of your life by asking others to pray for you and your spouse/partner, and you can do the same for them. You can post links to websites that you have found helpful and informative and learn what others have found in their search for knowledge. Some participants in online support groups use the strength of numbers to become politically active and lobby those in power for better access to services and treatments. Because of the anonymous nature of online support groups, you can also use this as a venue to vent safely—as long as your partner/spouse is not a participant of the same support group and you are venting about him!

WHICH SUPPORT GROUP IS RIGHT FOR ME?

You may be lucky enough to live in a city where there are multiple options for finding a support group that's right for you. But perhaps you live in a smaller city or town where there is just one support group for men with prostate cancer and their partners/spouses. You may go to a meeting and find that you really like it and continue to attend for months or even years. It's up to you. Or you may find that you don't like going or that the group doesn't meet your needs for support. That's also okay. You will read more about caring for yourself in the last chapter of this book, and self-care is very important if you are going to be able to support and care for your mate. Getting the support *you* need is an important aspect of self-care.

Before going to your first meeting, with your partner or by yourself, you may want to ask some questions about the group. Here is a list of questions to start the conversation:

- Who runs the group? Is it peer led (by someone with cancer or their spouse/partner), or is there a professional (for example a social worker or nurse) who leads the group?
- Is there a single facilitator, or do group members take turns?
- What is the focus of the group? Is it support or education or a combination of the two?
- What is the makeup of the group? How many men? Are women welcome? What about male partners? Are other family members welcome?
- Are men and their family members/spouses/partners split into separate groups for all or part of the meeting?
- What is the format of the meeting? How much time is allotted to education versus emotional support?
- Is there a fee associated with attendance?

There is no right or wrong answer to these questions, but you should get a feel for what the meetings are like from the way the person answers your questions. You may also have some ideas about what you are looking for—perhaps you would prefer the facilitator to be a professional, and if the group is peer led, you may want to think twice before committing. Or perhaps you can try one meeting and see how it goes.

WHAT COMES NEXT . . .

This book has mostly been about living and thriving in the world of prostate cancer. This is a very survivable cancer with a high rate of cure, but there are men who will die from this cancer. The next chapter talks about end-of-life care, a difficult subject to talk or even think about—but it is an important one because the end comes for all of us one day. That is just a reality of life. So take a deep breath and start reading if you want to. Or perhaps put that chapter aside and know that I hope you will never need to read it.

• *13* •

It All Went Wrong

End-of-Life Care

$\mathcal{D}$espite the very good cure rates and survival statistics for men with prostate cancer, some men will die of their disease. Even with the best efforts of the patient, his family, and the medical team, sometimes nothing can be done, and eventually the man runs out of treatment options. End-of-life issues must then be faced. This chapter will describe the end-of-life (or end-of-active-treatment) issues facing men with prostate cancer and their partners, with a focus on helping both of you cope with a sad reality.

It can happen; despite the really good odds that prostate cancer can be cured, some men will die of prostate cancer. Just 3 percent is the statistic most often quoted, but if your partner or spouse is one of the three in a hundred, nothing else matters. But how does it happen? To understand this, you need to go back to the beginning of this book where I explain about the need that prostate cancer has for the hormone testosterone. If there are any cancer cells left behind after surgery or radiation, in the presence of testosterone they will grow over time. Doctors will prescribe androgen deprivation therapy to starve those errant cells (as you read in chapter 9), but over time, the cancer cells become what is called "hormone" or "castrate" resistant; they grow despite being starved of testosterone.

CAN CHEMOTHERAPY BE USED?

There are still things that can be done if and when the man's cancer grows despite being starved of its fuel—chemotherapy has been shown to help with an increase in longevity of a couple of months (2.5 months). A drug called docetaxal is used with a steroid, and this has become the standard of care for men whose cancer has spread and does not respond to an absence of testosterone. It is usually given every three weeks, and about half of men getting this chemotherapy show a response with a drop in their PSA levels.[1] Other agents have been tested and for the most part have not achieved any better results. Docetaxal with steroids not only improved survival but also relieved pain and improved quality of life for men in the clinical trials. But there were also side effects, the most common being suppression of the bone marrow, leading to anemia (which makes men feel weak and tired), stomach upset, nerve pain, hair loss, and heart problems.

There are many other drugs being tested for men whose cancer continues to progress. Recent approvals from the FDA for a vaccine against the cancer that is made from the man's own immune cells in his blood (Sipuleucel-T) shows promise with a four-month increase in survival, but it comes at a large price (on average $93,000) and may not be available to all men because of where they live and proximity to facilities that can do the necessary procedures.[2] Another type of chemotherapy (called cabazitaxel) has also shown promise for men who have tried docetaxal before, with an additional 2.4 months of survival gained,[3] but this also has significant costs associated with it ($8,000 per cycle for a total of $48,000 for complete treatment). Another drug that seems hopeful is called abiraterone. It is not chemotherapy but rather a new kind of androgen deprivation therapy that prevents testosterone from being made in the body.[4] Men who took this drug lived for almost four months longer than those who took standard therapy, but once again, it is expensive, with a cost of $5,000 per cycle and a total cost of $40,000. There are many other treatments under study—I have not included them in this book because by the time you read this, some will have been shown to be of no use and others will be on the way to approval by the FDA.

It is important to note that most of these new agents are not only very expensive, but they also have significant side effects that are often not tolerated by men who are sick, especially those who are elderly. Aggressive treatment of hormone-resistant prostate cancer can itself cause death and will certainly reduce quality of life.[5] As with many other decisions about treatments, it is usually a question of balancing quality of life with length of life—and when you are facing the loss of someone you love dearly, this is very difficult if not impossible to do. The decision about the aggressiveness of treatment with small benefit is a very difficult one for all concerned—and sometimes the patient agrees to it because he can see how hard it is for his loved ones to "give up," but he may be tired and willing to forgo length of life for quality of life. But this may be hard for you to accept because you want him with you for as long as possible.

Norman had been an active participant in every aspect of his treatment since he was diagnosed more than eight years ago. He researched every treatment he was offered and at times his wife Rhoda wanted to burn the piles of papers, magazine articles, and books that were stacked (or scattered) all over their condo. But this was his way; he was a stubborn man, and he had to do things his way. She respected that and she loved him for it too. He had always been upbeat about his chances—but now the news was not good. She was confused by what he told her. He'd said that the cancer was back and that the injections he'd been having every six months for the last three years weren't working anymore.

"So try something else, Norm. There must be something else! What did your papers tell you?"

He just looked at her and shook his head. According to his doctors, there really was nothing else.

She sat in her favorite chair with a look of shock on her face. How could this be? She remembered what they had been told when he was first diagnosed.

"You'll die of something else, not the cancer!" were the words that the doctor had said, his voice confident and loud in the small office where they had waited to hear the results of the biopsy.

Had he lied? Why was Norman so willing to just accept this fate? He had to fight! He was a fighter! She would fight alongside him! But where to start?

WHAT IF ALL THE TREATMENTS DON'T WORK?

Some men will not respond to any of the established or experimental treatments for their cancer and will face the end of their life. And you will be by their side. How do you prepare for the death of someone you love? How do you face the end of the journey that you never wanted to see end? Let's start by talking about what happens when there are no more chances for cure of the cancer.

First, once all treatment options have been exhausted or the man with prostate cancer decides that he does not want anymore treatment, the focus of his care shifts from acute treatment to palliative care. Palliative care does not mean that the man is going to die soon, but rather that care now focuses on the man, his family, their attitudes and values, and his comfort, both physical and emotional. The target now is not cure or even control but rather providing him with what he needs to live with a chronic but terminal illness and to live the rest of his life as he wants to. The control now lies with the patient and his family and with their values and wishes for this next stage in his cancer journey.

This is a good time to make sure that you understand what his wishes are and to have these written down so that there is no confusion or reason for adult children or other relatives to question what is happening. The conversation can start with a single question: Where do you want to die? There are other questions of course: What, if any, medical intervention does he want? What does he want to happen if his heart stops beating? (Would he want CPR?) What if he gets an infection—does he want that to be treated with antibiotics or not? Who does he want to speak for him if he cannot speak for himself because he is in a coma? All of these directions should be written down in a document that is called a living will or advanced health-care directive. There are numerous examples of these documents online, but their legality is different depending on where you live, so it is best to talk to your health-care provider or lawyer about this. At its most basic, a living will or advanced health-care directive gives instructions about your wishes for treatment at the end of life should you not be able to speak for yourself. A health-care proxy (sometimes called a durable power of attorney) is a document that states who can make medical decisions for the patient should he not be able to speak for himself. While the man is still able to make decisions and speak for himself, health-care providers will seek his input about treatment decisions, but when he cannot do that, these documents play an important role in enacting his wishes.

WHAT HAPPENS AT THE END?

The man who has advanced prostate cancer and is approaching the end of his life will usually be weak and tired, and he will have lost a lot of weight. He may not be able to pass urine, as the tube that carries the urine out of the bladder may be blocked by cancer or enlarged lymph nodes. He may have swelling of the pelvic area and legs as a result of cancer in the lymph nodes of the pelvis. He may have anemia (low red cells in his blood), which leads to fatigue and shortness of breath as well as general weakness. He (and you) may feel depressed, anxious, and out of control.

Pain is very common at the end for many men with prostate cancer. Any cancer in his bones will continue to grow, and bone pain may be significant. This pain can impair his ability to get restful sleep, his appetite, and his desire to interact with people, including you and other loved ones. The importance of pain relief cannot be emphasized enough, and you should not worry that using powerful pain medication such as opioids (morphine and similar drugs) will lead to addiction as some people think. He needs long-acting pain medication to keep control over the pain for the long term, with some shorter-acting medications to control breakthrough pain. The doctor(s) treating his pain should strive to keep him as pain free as possible, but this may come at the price of his being very sleepy. The two of you have to decide what is most important—he may be willing to have some pain in order to be awake and aware of what is going on around him. On the other hand, he may wish to forgo that in order to be pain free.

If the cancer is in his spinal column, he may be at risk for something called *spinal cord compression*. This affects up to 12 percent of men with prostate cancer and is very serious.[6] Cancer in the bones of the spine can cause collapse of the vertebrae onto the spinal cord, or the cancer can grow into the space around the spinal cord and put pressure on the cord itself and the nerves that come out of the spinal cord. The onset of symptoms is usually slow, but it can also progress quite rapidly. Signs to look for that may indicate that something is wrong include increasing weakness or a feeling of heaviness in the feet and legs, severe pain in the back, and loss of bladder control. Emergency treatment is necessary, and this may include steroids, radiation to the area, or even surgery in some cases.[7]

Obstruction of the urethra can lead to urinary retention (inability to pass urine); this is painful and needs to be treated. For some men, insertion of a catheter into the bladder to relieve the pressure of the urine can be a great relief. The catheter may need to remain in place permanently, and often a decision is made to put the catheter into the bladder through the skin over the abdomen (called a suprapubic catheter) instead of through the penis. If the tubes that carry the urine from the kidneys to the bladder (the ureters) are blocked, small metal devices called stents can be placed into the tubes to keep them open and prevent the kidneys from being damaged.[8]

Lymphedema (swelling of the legs due to blockage or enlargement of the lymph glands) is often distressing to the man and his family and is often also painful and unsightly. Infection of the skin over the swollen area is not uncommon; this needs to be prevented if possible and treated promptly when it does occur. If the penis and scrotum become swollen, the pain may be quite severe; this may affect his ability to find a comfortable position, and he may need help moving in the bed. If you notice this swelling, call his doctor immediately.

There are specialized physiotherapists who may be able to provide a special kind of massage that promotes lymph drainage. Scrotal support is also necessary for comfort, but you need to be careful to not make the situation worse by compressing the area. Careful hygiene is important to prevent infection of the skin and also to provide comfort and help him feel better about himself. Lymphedema can impact self-esteem significantly, and many men with this condition tend to isolate themselves and refuse company. And of course this can then have an impact on you and your need for support from friends and family members.

Weight loss is very common in end-stage cancer of any kind, as the cancer uses a lot of energy to grow, and prostate cancer is no different. He may lose his *appetite*, and this also contributes to weight loss. Seeing him lose weight is distressing for family members, and it also plays a role in weakness and fatigue. There are medications that can increase his appetite, including megesterol acetate and steroids, but these have their own side effects. Along with loss of appetite, many men experience nausea. This may be a side effect of the pain medication or because the stomach and intestines slow down with lack of food and exercise. Antinausea medications can be used, but they also tend to make the man sleepy.

STAYING AT HOME OR GOING TO HOSPITAL OR HOSPICE

Gil and Tony had been together for what seemed to be forever, but now that Tony's journey with prostate cancer was coming to an end, there were not enough hours in the day for Gil. They had met when the AIDS crisis was at its peak, and they had watched friends and past lovers die of that terrible disease. Somehow they had both escaped that fate, and they felt so blessed that it had almost seemed impossible that anything bad was going to happen to either of them. But it had; Tony was diagnosed with advanced prostate cancer and just two short years later the time had come for him to face his final months. They'd talked about what they both wanted when he was first diagnosed; Gil wanted to take care of Tony at home, but Tony didn't want to burden him with that. They had both worked as volunteers at the Gay Men's Health Crisis Center in the old days, and they both knew what taking care of a dying person was like. Tony thought that it would be better if he went to a hospice or palliative care unit—he could get good care there and Gil could come and go. But Gil was having none of that. As soon as he saw how tired his beloved Tony was after going to the doctor's office the previous week, he went into full-on organizer mode. Within two days he had ordered a hospital bed from the medical supply store and had started calling around to their friends to set up a list of people to help with laundry and cooking and cleaning and shopping. It was like the 1980s had returned to their home—and Tony realized that he just had to go along with this for both their sakes.

Keeping the dying person at home for the final weeks and days of his life is a decision that is personal and hopefully is a decision that you should have discussed some time ago. Some people have very firm ideas about staying at home for these final days, but these same feelings are not reciprocated by their partner or spouse. Or your partner/spouse may not have decided what he wants to do and leaves that decision up to you. There is no right or wrong decision about this—you have to do what you are capable of and what you can bear. Some partners find great comfort in caring for their loved one at home in their final days, knowing that he is able to die in your own bed, or in a rented hospital bed in their own home. For other partners, the thought of witnessing his passage from life is scary and they don't want to think about sleeping in the same bed he died in. We are all different and will deal with this situation differently. But it's important to think about these things before they happen so that you can make the best decision for yourself in a thoughtful way instead of reacting to an emergency situation.

Of the men who die of prostate cancer in the United States each year, about half choose to die in a hospice.[9] Hospice care has been shown to improve quality of life at the end of life, quality of death, and symptom management. It also decreases the number of invasive and high-intensity but ultimately futile interventions that men receive at the end of life. Benefits of hospice care also include a homelike atmosphere and support for family with a personalized and individual focus so that your values and attitudes as a couple are respected more than in a hospital where the focus is on acute care and meeting goals for discharge.

WHAT WILL THE END LOOK LIKE?

Wherever your partner/spouse spends his final days and hours, you will have fears and concerns about what will happen. Many of us have not had the experience of seeing a loved one make the transition from life to death, and this fear can be overwhelming. Here is some general information about the end-of-life transition that may help prepare you, at least in part.

Most people at the end of life spend a lot of time sleeping, and it may be difficult to rouse him to eat or drink. The need for food and even water declines significantly in the last few days, and this is often a source of distress to family members who think that if they could only get some food or water into their loved one, things might improve. Forcing food or water on the dying person can be dangerous; he may inhale food or water into his lungs, which will cause choking. As death nears, the need for food and water goes away, and he will not feel hunger or even thirst. Keeping his lips moist with some lip balm or a wet cloth can be comforting to both of you.

Some people are also a little confused toward the end of life, and this can also be frightening for family members. The dying person may see things that are not there—a blanket may appear to him to be a dog or cat, for example. There is usually no point in trying to correct him; if he is distressed, remove the disturbing object and touch his arm or chest in a calm manner. This will help to sooth and comfort him, and he will drift off to sleep. Some dying people talk to people who are not in the room—their parents perhaps, or someone else who is no longer living. This can be a great comfort to him and to you—but it can also be distressing. You have to take things as they come, realize that this is an unpredictable time, and just do your best to be present for him while taking care of your own grief and sadness.

Even at the very end of life we think that people can hear what is said to them, so you may want to talk to your partner, even if he doesn't respond to you in a meaningful way. We cannot say with 100 percent certainty what he can hear or understand, but it will likely make you feel better to talk about what he has meant to you and to say your good-byes. Because he likely can hear, his bedside is not the place to have an argument with someone about funeral arrangements or issues related to money. And you may need to tell him that it is okay for him to "let go"—some people need permission to make that transition, and they often hang on because they are worried about you and how you will cope. Telling your partner that you will miss him but that you will be okay may be the permission that he needs to leave you, even though neither of you wants this. There are medications that can be used to sedate him and keep him in a deeper sleep, and you may want to talk to his health-care provider about using medication if either of you is distressed at this time. These medications are given to help avoid the confusion by keeping him asleep—they will not hasten death.

As his circulation shuts down, you may notice that his skin takes on a mottled appearance—his skin will look purplish and patchy, and his hands and feet will feel cool to the touch. This is a sign that death will come soon. His heart may beat faster, but it will be weak, and you may find it difficult to feel his pulse. His urinary system will also start to shut down, and if he has not been drinking he may not produce much urine. If he has not been eating, he may not have any bowel movements in the last few days.

As his last hours near, you will notice changes in his breathing; these can be distressing because to you it may seem as if he is struggling for breath, but in fact the changes I'm going to describe are normal at the end of life. He may start using the muscles in his neck to breathe, and this may lift his shoulder slightly. This is not a sign of a struggle for breath, but rather the automatic centers of the brain taking over. He may also make noises, like snoring, when he breathes. This is due to a buildup of fluids in his throat and lungs, and though he is not aware of it (just like snoring!) it can be awful for you to hear it. There are medications that can help with this; they are given by a patch on the skin or by injection and can be helpful. He will also breathe in a more mechanical way, and his breaths will become more shallow and rapid, and then he will have some pauses in his breathing. These pauses may last as long as thirty seconds and may be distressing to you, but this is normal and is usually a good indication that death will come soon. In the final hours or minutes of his life, his breathing will become irregular, with one or two breaths, then a pause, then perhaps another breath followed by a pause, and so forth. You may find yourself holding your breath when he doesn't breathe, and then only being able to breathe again when he takes a breath.

And then finally that pause will lengthen, and he will not take another breath. It may be hard for you to tell what has happened. He may make a few, small reflex movements, but he will not take another breath. It is over. You will not be able to see or feel a pulse in his neck or at his wrists. His eyes will close, partway or fully, and his pupils will be large and dark and they will not react to a light shining into them. If you are in a hospice or hospital, staff will be close by to help you realize that the end has come. It is not easy, but it has happened, and now your mourning work starts.

AND AFTER THE END?

There is no hurry to "do something" once he is gone. You may sit with him, talk with him, and touch him until you are ready to say your final good-bye. There is also no "right" way to react, act, or feel. You may be relieved that his suffering and pain are over. You may feel guilty that you are relieved. You may feel shock that this has happened even though you were prepared for it. You may not have been in the room at the moment of death—perhaps you went to get something to drink—and this can cause you to feel guilty that you "missed it"; it is common for the dying person to somehow wait for their loved ones to leave the room before they let go and die. We're not sure why this happens, or even how, but it is something that is quite common.

Hopefully the two of you discussed any wishes that he had about burial or cremation, a service or remembrance ceremony, or any other details that are important now that he is gone. You don't have to hurry to organize any of this—but it may feel good to have something to do in the first few days. This is also a good time to get family and friends to help you with driving, getting food in the house, and so forth. They want to help, and if you tell them what to do, you will make them feel useful. This will also allow you to take the time you need to let this settle into your new life without his presence.

⸺⁓◦◦◦⁓⸺

Ramone had slipped out of life just the way that he lived it; it was quiet in the room where Sofia sat with her head resting on the edge of his bed. She must have dozed off because when she opened her eyes, she was aware that there was no sound other than her own breathing.

She went cold all over and stared at the face of the man she loved above all else. His face was still, so still, and his eyes were half closed. She knew it when she looked in his eyes; they didn't shine back at her, their surface was dull, as if someone had dried his eyes with a cloth.

She felt a scream rise up in her throat, and she put her hands over her mouth to keep the sound in. Her heart was beating really fast and for an awful moment she thought that she might throw up. Her hand was shaking as she reached for the call bell that was pinned to the pillow close to where his hand, now so cold, lay on the sheet. She needed a nurse or a doctor to help her—where were they? Why were they not in the room? Why did they not do something? Before she pushed the red button, she heard the door open quietly and the voice of Stella, the nurse:

"Sofia, are you okay?"

Sofia was definitely not okay, and this time she couldn't hold the sound back; she let it go, a wail that could be heard all the way down the hallway and out into the street.

HOW DO YOU COPE WITH ALL OF THIS?

In the next chapter you will read about the importance of taking care of yourself and how to seek and accept help. After your partner/spouse dies, your need for support does not diminish and may increase; if you feel like it, reach out to family and friends who love you and want to help in whatever way they can.

We all mourn in different ways, and no one should tell you how to feel or how to be. Don't add to your burden by thinking that there is a right way or a wrong way to act or feel, or that there is some prescribed timeline for "getting over" this. Some people find that clearing out their partner's closet is a good distraction in the days following his passing, while others think that it is too soon to do that (and the time may never be right!). Others need to nestle down in their home and just let their emotions take over. They may feel sad and cry for weeks or months or even longer. Some partners have to go back to work soon after the funeral or service, and it is always surprising to hear that some companies expect a bereaved spouse to return to work within forty-eight hours of a partner's death.

WHAT COMES NEXT . . .

This may have been a difficult chapter to read—and it was not easy to write! Talking and thinking about death is not easy, and it is my fervent hope that no one needs to read this chapter—although of course there are some of you who must read it because you are faced with end-of-life issues for your spouse or partner. The next chapter focuses on *you*—it is about self-care and the need to look after your own health, physical and emotional, so that you can help your partner face all of the challenges and triumphs of life in general, and life with prostate cancer specifically.

RESOURCES

http://www.virtualhospice.ca/en_US/Main+Site+Navigation/Home.aspx
> The Canadian Virtual Hospice website is a comprehensive website for information about end-of-life issues that are universal and not just for Canadians.

http://www.cancer.gov/cancertopics/factsheet/Support/palliative-care
> This website, part of the National Cancer Institute, provides information about palliative care for people with cancer.

http://familydoctor.org/familydoctor/en/diseases-conditions/cancer/treatment/palliative-care.html
> This is another website that gives general information about palliative care from the American Academy of Family Physicians.

http://www.hospicedirectory.org
> The Hospice Foundation of America sponsors this website, which has information about hospice care, including a useful feature to find a hospice where you live.

http://www.nahc.org/haa/about.html

The Hospice Association of America is a national organization representing thousands of hospices, caregivers, and volunteers who serve terminally ill patients and their families. This is primarily a lobby group and does not provide direct service but rather represents hospices across the United States.

Don't Worry about Me!

Self-Care

$\mathcal{H}$ow do you take care of yourself in the midst of caring for him? How do you cope with stress while trying to take care of those around you? Where can you go for help when you feel overwhelmed or tired or out of control? These questions and more will be answered in this chapter.

This is the last chapter in the book—but it really should have been the first. If you don't take care of yourself, you really can't take care of, or take part in the care of, your partner or spouse. But so often we forget this and put everyone else's needs before our own, and we end up not being able to help anyone. In some cases we get sick physically or emotionally, and then we really can't help him.

There are some general things to do to take care of yourself—getting enough sleep, eating well, finding time to exercise, and asking for and accepting help and support—but there are also things that you need to do that relate to the fact that your spouse/partner has been diagnosed with cancer. So let's look at the ways in which you can take care of yourself, and as a result be able to take care of your spouse/partner, that are specific to his prostate cancer journey.

GENERAL SELF-CARE

Paula felt like a truck had hit her. Ever since they had found out about Harvey's cancer it had been a whirlwind of doctors' appointments and tests and scans. She had spent more time in waiting rooms in the past three weeks than she had in all her life. She was not a patient person at the best of times, and the wasted time was

171

getting to her. She knew that it didn't help Harvey when she got all worked up, but at times it was hard for her to keep her mouth shut. She was really worried about the outcome of all the tests, and the thought of losing Harvey was too much for her.

She felt like she hadn't slept in weeks, and when she thought about it, she really hadn't had a good night's sleep since they heard the news. She fell asleep on the couch most nights and then struggled to get to sleep when she went to bed. She would then wake up two or three hours later and start to think about the cancer, and that was pretty much it for the rest of the night. She hadn't been able to go for her daily walk either because she didn't want to leave his side. She knew this was silly, but she had to keep him close all the time. Her usually short temper and low tolerance for things were at an all-time low; just yesterday she almost yelled at the young man who was bagging her groceries. He'd put the dairy in with the vegetables, and she could feel her anger like a red hot wave, rising toward her mouth. She'd looked at Harvey, and he had this look on his face like he wanted the floor to swallow him. She'd managed to take a deep breath and stop herself from yelling, but it was close.

SLEEP: THE GREAT HEALER

Many of us don't get enough sleep. Our need for sleep seems to change as we get older, but we still have a basic need not only for adequate sleep but also for sleep of good quality. Many women find that their sleep quality declines during and after menopause. This is not just something that you have to accept—if you are not getting restful sleep because of hot flashes and night sweats, do something about it! Many of the suggestions I am going to make in the following pages may help—but you should also talk to your primary care or women's health provider to see if there is something else that can help. An exhausted person is not much good to anyone.

Here are some suggestions that may help you improve your sleep:

- Keep to a regular sleep-wake schedule. Go to bed at the same time and get up at the same time as much as possible.
- Create a bedtime routine that signals to your brain that sleep is coming and it should wind down. Having something warm to drink (avoid caffeine and alcohol), a warm bath or shower, or listening to soft music is a good place to start. A simple action like rubbing lotion into your hands as you prepare to sleep or meditating can also be useful—and both of these activities feel good and are good for you.
- If you are sensitive to caffeine or alcohol, avoid drinking or eating them (chocolate contains caffeine) from midafternoon on.

- Try not to nap too late in the afternoon and absolutely not in the evening. If you are falling asleep watching TV at night, it means that you need to go to bed and get some restful sleep.
- Make the room as dark as you can with blackout blinds and turn your LED alarm clock toward the wall; even that small amount of light can disturb your sleep.
- Try not to watch TV in bed—this is hard, I know, but the light from the screen stimulates the brain, and the content of the news or drama shows interferes with restful and restorative sleep.
- If you can't fall asleep, avoid watching TV. Get up, go to another room, and read under a soft light for a while. When you feel tired, go back to bed and lie quietly in the dark.
- If you wake during the night, follow the instructions for falling asleep—no TV, read in a dim light, and go back to bed when you feel sleepy.
- Deep and regular breathing can help you get to sleep too. Repeat as often as necessary until you actually do fall asleep.
- Try to address your worries before you go to bed. Talk about them to someone who is part of your support system or even write them down; this can take them off your mind and allow you to fall asleep instead of lying there and worrying. Do the same with things you have to do the next day or week—make a list and let go of the need to remember.

NOURISH YOUR BODY

Merrill's best friend said it first, but she could see that the rest of her friends were thinking it too.

"Good grief, Merrill! You look like one of those super skinny models—and that isn't a compliment! What on earth have you done to yourself?"

Merrill couldn't answer at first. She tried to speak, but instead of words, a sob came out of her mouth. She sat down quickly, put her hands over her face, and let the tears come. Her friends all rushed to her side, patting her back and murmuring her name, but it felt good to cry, especially after she'd been holding back the tears for so long.

She knew she looked drawn—who wouldn't after what she'd gone through—and her clothes didn't fit right anymore. But who could eat when your husband was going to the hospital every day for those radiation treatments? Most of the time she felt sick to her stomach, and on the odd occasion when she felt hungry, she was either in the car or waiting for him to be done. He just wanted toast for dinner most nights, and so she had some with him and they went to bed. He was that wiped out. And so was she. But what else could she do? She had to put him first, and she was doing just that.

———— ✺ ————

You need to take care of your body, and that means giving it the right kind of fuel to do its work. Many of us don't eat properly when we are stressed or busy. We grab food on the fly, eat it without being aware of what and how much we are eating, and as a result eat things that are not good for us even though they are readily available. These are often packaged foods, heavy on the carbohydrates and fat and low on protein and fiber. It's easier to throw a muffin into your bag than an egg, and there are always packages of cookies at the cash register when you buy your to-go cup of coffee or tea. They fill you up, raise your blood sugar, and then an hour or so later, your blood sugar drops and you need something else to eat. So you repeat the actions above. Sitting in waiting rooms while your partner/spouse has tests or treatments or recovers from surgery is boring, but you may not want to leave the area—and so you subsist on coffee from a vending machine, a chocolate bar, or a bag of nacho chips.

So how can you eat well and nourish your body so that it can do what it needs to? Make the effort to fuel your body with the best-quality food you can give it, being mindful that you probably don't have the time or energy to cook gourmet foods. The point is that you don't have to! Here are some general suggestions that may help.

- When your friends ask what they can do for you, tell them that you would appreciate some meals in one- or two-serving helpings that you can freeze for eating later or heat up quickly in the microwave. And then eat them!
- Ask your friends to go to the grocery store for you. They want to help, so ask them for some specific help instead of just saying, "Oh, I'm fine."
- Keep fresh fruits in the fridge and on the kitchen counter and eat whole fruits rather than drinking fruit juice. You'll consume less added sugar and more fiber. Fruit comes in nature's own wrapper, so keep a banana, orange, or apple in your bag or car, and you'll always have something healthy to snack on.
- Try to eat some protein with every meal, and if you have a protein-based snack, you'll be less likely to snack on high-calorie sweet things. A hard-boiled egg is easy to grab and take with you. Cheese is easily

transportable too and will survive an hour or more outside the fridge. A handful of almonds is highly nutritious and satisfying because you have to chew and not just swallow!

- Yogurt is also great to eat in a hurry—add some granola for extra crunch or dip a banana into the container. Greek yogurt has a good amount of protein in it, and if you buy the plain kind and add fruit to it, you can avoid added sugars entirely.
- Try to sit down to eat rather than standing at the kitchen counter or in front of the fridge. And when you do eat, just do that. No TV, no book, no newspaper. Being mindful and actually thinking about the food in your mouth and in your stomach is much more beneficial than eating mindlessly with distractions.
- Be careful about filling up with soda, tea, or coffee. None of these contains much nutrition, and while they may stop the hunger pangs for a short time, they do not provide the sustenance that your body needs.
- All this healthy eating doesn't mean that you can't have chocolate ever—just be judicious about eating well most of the time, and having a treat, and really enjoying it, is part of eating well.

STRESS RELIEF = EXERCISE

You've heard it a million times before—exercise is good for you. And you may even believe it! But exercise is not only good for your body—it's good for your mind and soul too. Exercise can help with mild to moderate depression, and when combined with its other beneficial effects, it will improve your overall quality of life. But there are times when making the effort to find the time to exercise just seems overwhelming. Here are some suggestions to get you moving:

- Promise yourself that you will do just ten minutes of exercise every day. Once you get going, you will find that it is easy to continue beyond the ten minutes because you actually enjoy it.
- Forgive yourself if you don't exercise every day—but get right back to your plans as soon as possible before you lose motivation.
- Do something you know you can do—everyone can walk if they are able.
- Exercise with a friend and use the time to reconnect or get support. Having a responsibility to a friend also means that you're less likely to not do what you planned.

- Your partner can be your exercise buddy as his recovery permits. He needs exercise for all the same reasons you do. But you also deserve a break from him and your caregiving duties, so think about who you want to exercise with.
- Wear the right clothes for the activity. Being incorrectly dressed can make your efforts feel uncomfortable, and then you are more likely to give it up.
- Don't make unrealistic plans—running a marathon in two months' time is not realistic.

CANCER SELF-CARE

"What if?": Dealing with Fears and Feelings

Alexander had never dealt well with stressful situations, and Galen had always been the one to support him if anything went wrong. But now it was Galen who had "gone wrong," and Alexander didn't know who to turn to for support. He felt so alone ever since Galen had been diagnosed with prostate cancer, and he didn't know where to turn. It was worse at night when the apartment was quiet. Galen slept soundly, and Alexander paced the three rooms outside their bedroom. Back and forth he went, barefoot so that he wouldn't wake his partner. It seemed as if a new worry popped into his head with each turn he made.

He had lots to worry about: Galen was the breadwinner, and he'd been off work for five weeks since the surgery. He was also the only one with a driver's license, so Alexander had to get on the bus to buy groceries and go to the drugstore. But mostly Alexander was scared about Galen. They were going to the doctor the following week to hear if they had gotten all the cancer out during the operation, and Alexander was in a panic. What if there was cancer left behind? What more could they do for him? Why didn't they just give him chemo now and avoid trouble later? How was he going to cope if Galen needed to go to the hospital every day? Galen himself seemed to not be worried at all. But all Alexander could think about was all the things that could go wrong.

When faced with the diagnosis of a serious illness in someone you love (and cancer is about as serious as it gets), it may be difficult if not impossible to keep fears in check. Playing the "what-if" game is common—What if he dies? What if I'm left alone? What if we can't afford the recommended treatment? What if his cancer comes back? What if he has pain? These are all important questions—but endlessly thinking about them and not doing anything to quiet those fears is futile. Many people play the "what-if" game late at night when they're trying to go to sleep. The questions swirl in your head, and each unanswered question makes your heart beat faster and your mouth get dry. And sleep doesn't come, so you have even more time to think of additional "what-if" questions.

It is important to talk about what you are afraid of, because just in talking about it the fears are often tamed, or at least made smaller and more manageable. And let your partner/spouse in on your feelings—he is equally worried about the same issues and is, like you, trying to protect the person he loves most. Naming the fear helps you to deal with what you are afraid of and takes away the power that the fear has on your life. Talk about your fear of being left alone; he is thinking the same thing and may feel guilty about having cancer because of this. In talking about it, you will realize how much support you have—perhaps from your children or extended family and friends—and you will begin to anticipate how you will use their love and support to help you feel less alone if and when your spouse/partner reaches the end of his life. After treatment, your partner, like you, is certainly worried about the cancer coming back; almost all cancer survivors experience this fear of recurrence. But he may be afraid to talk to you about it because he doesn't want to worry you—but you are doing a fine job of worrying on your own! Talking about the fear may lead to the two of you finding out the real statistics about cancer recurrence and hopefully understanding the real risks, which may be much smaller than you assume. There's an old saying about a problem shared being a problem halved, and that is often true. You are in this together, and you will find your way out of the "what-if" together too.

If you have religious faith, you may be able to share your worries with a priest, rabbi, imam, pastor, or other religious leader. Putting your experience into the bigger picture and finding meaning is one of the unexpected benefits of facing a life-threatening illness personally or in someone you love. Cancer survivors and their partners have talked about this eloquently in many studies, and finding meaning in the cancer journey may take you to a place in your life that is much richer than where you were when the journey first started.[1] And finding meaning does not have to come from formal religious ritual and practice. You can find that meaning in talking and thinking and journaling about what has happened and how it has changed you.

Being in the moment may also help. Fears and anxieties are future oriented—"What will happen if . . . ?" is about something that has not occurred. Being focused on what is in the here and now instead of what might happen in the future can be a helpful strategy for managing fear. Mindfulness practice is something that you might want to think about. While not a religion at all, it is based on Buddhist philosophy and has been shown to be effective in helping patients with cancer and other diseases deal with the stress of illness and the uncertainty of the future. There are a number of books on the subject, as well as tapes and CDs that provide guidance for doing mindfulness meditation. These resources are listed at the end of the chapter. By being focused on the present, you can deal with reality instead of worrying about something that has not happened or may never happen.

DENIAL IS NOT JUST A RIVER IN EGYPT

There are times when denying that something is happening is protective. Thinking or pretending that your partner doesn't have cancer or isn't going to die can help in a way if it allows you to be positive and to have the energy to find the answers you need. But denial can also mean that you do nothing, and that is not good. If denial stops you from finding out information or taking in the information that health-care professionals are telling you, it's time to leave that river in Egypt and get on the reality train.

Denial is also different from the shock you experience when you first hear the words "I have cancer" coming out of the mouth of your partner. That shock may prevent you from hearing anything else in the short term. It may also cause your heart to beat faster and your breath to almost stop. But that shock is and should be a temporary thing, and once you have recovered from the immediacy of that physical and emotional reaction, you need to get into action mode so that you can help your partner and yourself get started on the journey through understanding about the cancer, doing something about treatment when necessary, and then moving with him into the world of cancer survivorship, where hopefully you will live for a long time.

GETTING ANGRY

Tina and Gerald had only been married for three years when he was diagnosed with prostate cancer; he was twenty years older than she was, and her mother had warned her that marrying an older man would mean that she was going to have to nurse him sooner rather than later. Tina had laughed it off at the time—but her mother's prediction, cruel as it was, had come true. He was sixty years old, but the surgery and then the radiation had turned him into an old man.

He'd promised her twenty good years—years of travel and theater and great restaurants and adventures. She'd gotten three years of good times, but the two years since his treatment had not been good at all. He was not the man she had married, and they were not the couple she had thought they would be. He wanted to stay home most of the time, and she understood that it was difficult for him to go out because he needed to be close to a restroom at all times. She knew he was in pain most of the time, and she felt bad about that. But he was the one who wouldn't take his pain pills. He was grumpy, and they'd started sleeping in separate rooms because he was up half the night. She was only forty-five, and she felt that she had been cheated out of a lot. She was angry at him, and angry at the cancer, and angry at what her life had become. It was just not fair!

It's not uncommon to experience anger when faced with the illness of a loved one. It's not fair that this has happened to both of you, and you have every right to be angry about it. But you need to be careful about where and how you express that anger—and especially careful about being angry at *him* rather than at the cancer. This doesn't mean that you have to be something that you are not—being an all-forgiving angel is difficult, and the things that he usually does that irritate or anger you are still going to be there. But the anger you feel at the cancer should not be directed at him.

You may be angry at health-care providers who don't seem to be listening or doing enough or taking enough time to meet your needs. You may be angry with your children, who are busy with their lives and not being supportive enough. Or with friends who don't seem to know what to do or how to help. You may also be angry at the things you have to do that your partner used to do but now can't. And you may be angry at yourself for not coping as well as you think you should, or for crying, or for feeling depressed. There is no "right" way to be or feel or cope—you are doing the best you can in a situation in which you have no control and absolutely no training. Be careful of bottling up your emotions (anger, sadness, fear, or guilt), because not dealing with emotion can have significant and negative effects on your health. You may find that you start to have physical symptoms yourself—headaches, stomach pains, a rash, or panic attacks to name just a few—and while these are real, the reason for them is that you are not dealing with the stress of the illness, and the bottled-up emotions are finding a way to get out.

Find a safe place to express your anger at what has happened: a supportive friend, a support group for partners of people with cancer, or a counselor or therapist. Writing down your feelings can help too—and burning or otherwise destroying the pages can be a powerful symbol of letting your anger go. Everyone has different ways of experiencing and expressing their anger, but dealing with it in a constructive manner and then moving on and away from it is what's important.

GETTING HELP

If you can't deal with your feelings and fears, and if you are feeling depressed and anxious to the point that you can't do what you need to do in your day, then you may need professional help. It's nothing to be ashamed of, and yet seeking help is often seen to be a sign of weakness and a source of shame. If you broke your arm, you wouldn't try to fix it yourself or walk around in pain, unable to brush your teeth or make a cup of coffee, would you? So why is it so hard to get help when our heart is broken or our brain is full of worry and fear?

Some people find that talking to a friend is helpful—but a friend can only do so much, and it may not be fair to burden a friend with something that he or she can't cope with effectively because they are a friend and not a professional. There is help available to you as the partner/spouse of a man with cancer—most cancer centers and hospitals have social workers (sometimes called "psychosocial clinicians"), psychologists, psychiatrists, and counselors to provide support to both patients and their families. Your primary care provider may also help—and will be able to refer you to other professionals if necessary.

Attending a support group for partners of people with cancer can also be helpful. Hearing how other people in a similar situation cope can be enlightening, and being able to share your feelings with others who are "walking the same walk" may even be better for you than talking to a professional. But remember that these are people just like you, and they shouldn't be telling you what to do, how to feel, or how to react. The emphasis of a support group is on support, not on treating or managing someone else's emotional or physical health.

WHAT COMES NEXT . . .

This is the final chapter of this book. So what comes next is in your hands. I hope that you have learned about prostate cancer and how it affects both of you in a way that is meaningful to you. A lot of ground has been covered over the past fourteen chapters, and in many ways you are now an expert in prostate cancer from a partner's perspective. This will allow you to be a full player in your partner's care should you choose to do that. One of the first statements in this book is that prostate cancer is a couple's disease—you may not have realized that when you started reading, but I hope that you know and believe it now.

RESOURCES ON MINDFULNESS

Letting Everything Become Your Teacher: 100 Lessons in Mindfulness, by Jon Kabat Zinn (Delta Publishing, 2009).

Arriving at Your Own Door: 108 Lessons in Mindfulness, by Jon Kabat Zinn (Hyperion, 2007).

Mindfulness for Beginners, by Jon Kabat Zinn (CD; Sounds True Inc., 2006).

Coming to Our Senses: Healing Ourselves and the World through Mindfulness, by Jon Kabat Zinn (Hyperion, 2006).

Wherever You Go, There You Are, by Jon Kabat Zinn (Hyperion, 2005).

Full Catastrophe Living: Using the Wisdom of Your Body and Mind to Face Stress, Pain, and Illness, by Jon Kabat Zinn (Delta Publishing, 1990).

Guided Mindfulness Meditation, by Jon Kabat Zinn (CD; Sounds True Inc., 2005).

Notes

CHAPTER 1

1. D. Eton, S. LePore, and V. Helgeson. (2005). Psychological distress in spouses of men treated for early-stage prostate carcinoma. *Cancer, 103*, 2412–2418.
2. G. Bodenmann. (2005). Dyadic coping and its significance for marital functioning. In T. A. Revenson, K. Kayser, & G. Bodenmann (Eds.), *Couples coping with stress: Emerging perspectives on dyadic coping* (pp. 33–49). Washington, DC: American Psychological Association.
3. Morgan, M. (2009). Considering the patient-partner relationship in cancer care: Coping strategies for couples. *Clinical Journal of Oncology Nursing, 13*(1), 65–72.
4. G. Perlman and J. Drescher. (2005). *A gay man's guide to prostate cancer*. Binghamton, NY: Haworth Medical Press; G. Perlman. (2012). *What every gay man needs to know about prostate cancer: The essential guide to diagnosis, treatment, and recovery.* New York: Magnus Books.
5. T. Tanner, M. Galbraith, and L. Hays. (2011). From a woman's perspective: Life as a partner of a prostate cancer survivor. *Journal of Midwifery and Women's Health, 56*, 154–160.
6. B. Davison, M. Gleave, S. Goldenberg, L. Degner, D. Hoffart, and J. Berkowitz. (2002). Assessing information and decision preferences of men with prostate cancer and their partners. *Cancer Nursing, 25*, 42–49.

CHAPTER 2

1. D. Arnold-Reed, D. Hince, M. Bulsara, H. Ngo, M. Eaton, A. Wrights, et al. Knowledge and attitudes of men about prostate cancer. *MJA, 189*(6), 312–314.
2. B. Miles, B. Giesler, and M. Kattan. (1999). Recall and attitudes in patients with prostate cancer. *Urology, 53*, 169–174.

183

3. F. Fowler, M. Barry, B. Walker-Corkery, J. Caubet, D. Bates, J. Min Lee, et al. (2006). The impact of a suspicious prostate biopsy on patients' psychological, socio-behavioral, and medical care outcomes. *Journal of General Internal Medicine, 21*, 715–721.

4. L. Resendes and R. McCorkle. (2006). Spousal responses to prostate cancer: An integrative review. *Cancer Investigation, 24*, 192–198.

5. S. Roesch, L. Adams, A. Hines, A. Palmores, P. Vyas, C. Tran, et al. (2005). Coping with prostate cancer: A meta-analytic review. *Journal of Behavioral Medicine, 28*(3), 281–293.

6. I. Korfage, H. de Koning, M. Roobol, F. Schroder, and M. Essink-Bot. (2006). Prostate cancer diagnosis: The impact on patients' mental health. *European Journal of Cancer, 42*, 165–170.

7. N. Awsare, J. Green, B. Aldwinckle, D. Hanbury, G. Boustead, and R. McNicholas. (2008). The measurement of psychological distress in men being investigated for the presence of prostate cancer. *Prostate Cancer and Prostatic Diseases, 11*, 384–389.

8. C. Sharpley, D. Christie, and V. Bitsika. (2010). Variability in anxiety and depression over time following diagnosis in patients with prostate cancer. *Journal of Psychosocial Oncology, 28*, 644–665.

9. K. Fall, F. Fang, L. Mucci, W. Ye, O. Andren, J. Johansson, et al. (2009). Immediate risk for cardiovascular events and suicide following a prostate cancer diagnosis: Prospective cohort study. *PLos Medicine, 6*: e1000197.doi:10.1371/journal .pmed.1000197.

10. L. Northouse, D. Mood, A. Schafenacker, J. Montie, H. Sandler, J. Forman, et al. (2007). Randomized clinical trial of a family intervention for prostate cancer patients and their spouses. *Cancer, 110*, 2809–2818.

11. R. Gray, M. Fitch, C. Phillips, M. Labrecque, and K. Fergus. (2000). To tell or not to tell: Patterns of disclosure among men with prostate cancer. *Psycho-Oncology, 9*, 273–282.

CHAPTER 3

1. F. Fowler, M. McNaughton Collins, P. Albertsen, A. Zietman, D. Elliott, and M. Barry. (2000). Comparison of recommendations by urologists and radiation oncologists for treatment of localized prostate cancer. *JAMA, 283*(4), 3217–3222.

2. D. Feldman-Stewart, M. Brundage, C. Hayter, J. Davidson, P. Groome, and J. Nickel. (1997). What the prostate cancer patient should know: Variations in urologists' opinions. *Canadian Journal of Urology, 4*(4), 438–444.

3. R. Chen, J. Clark, J. Manola, and J. Talcott. (2008). Treatment "mismatch" in early prostate cancer: Do treatment choices take patient quality of life into account? *Cancer, 112*, 61–68.

4. F. Joudi and B. Konety. (2005). The impact of provider volume on outcomes from urological cancer therapy. *Journal of Urology, 174*, 432–438.

5. J. Hoffman, M. Wilkes, F. Fay, F. Bell, and J. Higa. (2006). The roulette wheel: An aid to informed decision making. *PLoS Medicine, 3*(6), 743–748.

6. V. Nanton and J. Dale. (2009). Prostate cancer: Balancing the need to inform with the patient's wish to know. *BJU International, 103*, 1603–1605.

7. M. Politi and R. Street. (2010). The importance of communication in collaborative decision making: Facilitating shared mind and the management of uncertainty. *Journal of Evaluation in Clinical Practice.* doi:10.1111/j.1365-2753.2010.01549.x

8. S. Shariat, P. Karakiewicz, C. Roehrborn, and M. Kattan. (2008). An updated catalog of prostate cancer predictive tools. *Cancer, 113*, 3075–3099.

9. T. Yap, J. Armitage, M. Emberton, and J. Ven Den Meulen. (2006). Information booklets for men with localized prostate cancer need to be improved. *BJU International, 98*(2), 251–252.

10. D. Stacey, R. Samant, and C. Bennett. (2008). Decision making in oncology: A review of patient decision aids to support patient participation. *CA: A Cancer Journal for Clinicians, 58*, 293–304.

11. G. Lin, D. Aaronson, S. Knight, P. Carroll, and A. Dudley. (2009). Patient decision aids for prostate cancer treatment: A systematic review of the literature. *CA: A Journal for Clinicians, 59*, 379–390.

12. J. van den Meulen, J. Jansen, J. van Dulmen, J. Bensing, and J. van Weert. (2008). Interventions to improve recall of medical information in cancer patients: A systematic review of the literature. *Psycho-Oncology, 17*, 857–868.

13. N. Henrikson, W. Ellis, and D. Berry. (2009). "It's not like I can change my mind later": Reversibility and decision timing in prostate cancer treatment decision-making. *Patient Education and Counseling, 77*, 302–307.

14. S. Zeliadt, S. Ramsey, D. Penson, I. Hall, D. Ekwueme, L. Stroud, and J. Lee. (2006). Why do men choose one treatment over another? A review of patient decision making for localized prostate cancer. *Cancer, 106*, 1865–1874.

15. B. Sommers, C. Beard, A. D'Amico, I. Kaplan, J. Richie, and R. Zeckhauser. (2008). Predictors of patient preferences and treatment choices for localized prostate cancer. *Cancer, 113*, 2058–2067.

16. S. Zeliadt, C. Moinpour, D. Blough, D. Penson, I. Hall, J. Smith, et al. (2010). Preliminary treatment considerations among men with newly diagnosed prostate cancer. *American Journal of Managed Care, 16*(5): e121–e130.

17. S. Steginga, E. Turner, and J. Donovan. (2008). The decision-related psychosocial concerns of men with localized prostate cancer: Targets for intervention and research. *World Journal of Urology, 26*, 469–474.

18. H. Orom, L. Penner, B. West, T. Downs, and W. Rayford. (2009). Personality predicts prostate cancer treatment decision-making difficulty and satisfaction. *Psycho-Oncology, 18*, 290–299.

19. M. Walsh, A. Trentham-Dietz, T. Schroepfer, D. Reding, B. Campbell, M. Foote, et al. (2010). Cancer information sources used by patients to inform and influence treatment decisions. *Journal of Health Communication, 15*, 445–463.

20. S. Ramsey, S. Zeliadt, N. Arora, A. Potosky, D. Blough, A. Hamilton, et al. (2009). Access to information sources and treatment considerations among men with local stage prostate cancer. *Urology, 74*, 509–516.

21. C. Lee, S. Gray, and N. Lewis. (2010). Internet use leads cancer patients to be active health care consumers. *Patient Education and Counseling, 81S*, S63–S69.

22. W. Underwood, H. Orom, M. Poch, B. West, P. Lantz, S. Chang, and J. Fowke. (2010). Multiple physician recommendations for prostate cancer treatment: A Pandora's box for patients? *Canadian Journal of Urology, 17*(5), 5346–5354.

23. C. Gwede, J. Pow-Sang, J. Seigne, R. Heysek, M. Helal, K. Shade, et al. (2005). Treatment decision-making strategies and influences in patients with localized prostate cancer. *Cancer, 104*, 1381–1390.

24. M. Diefenbach and N. Mohamed. (2007). Regret of treatment decision and its association with disease-specific quality of life following prostate cancer treatment. *Cancer Investigation, 25*, 449–457.

25. T. Denberg, B. Beaty, F. Kim, and J. Steiner. (2005). Marriage and ethnicity predict treatment in localized prostate carcinoma. *Cancer, 103*, 1819–1825.

26. Henrikson, Ellis, and Berry. (2009).

27. B. Davison, L. Goldenberg, M. Gleave, and L. Degner. (2003). Provision of individualized information to men and their partners to facilitate treatment decision making in prostate cancer. *Oncology Nursing Forum, 30*(1), 107–114.

28. K. Echlin and C. Rees. (2002). Information needs and information-seeking behaviors of men with prostate cancer and their partners: A review of the literature. *Cancer Nursing, 25*(1), 35–41.

29. K. Schumm, Z. Skea, L. McKee, and J. N'Dow. (2010). "They're doing surgery on two people": A meta-ethnography of the influences on couples' treatment decision making for prostate cancer. *Health Expectations, 13*, 335–349.

30. D. Zwhalen, N. Hagenbuch, M. Carley, J. Jenewein, and S. Buchi. (2010). Posttraumatic growth in cancer patients and partners: Effects of role, gender and the dyad on couples' posttraumatic growth experience. *Psycho-Oncology, 19*, 12–20.

31. S. Maliski, M. Hellemann, and R. McCorkle. (2002). From "death sentence" to "good cancer": Couples' transformation of a prostate cancer diagnosis. *Nursing Research, 51*(6), 391–397.

CHAPTER 4

1. L. Klotz. (2008). Low-risk prostate cancer can and should often be managed with active surveillance and selective delayed intervention. *Nature Clinical Practice Urology, 5*(1), 2–3.

2. J. Hayes, D. Ollendorf, S. Pearson, M. Barry, P. Kantoff, S. Stewart, et al. (2010). Active surveillance compared with initial treatment for men with low-risk prostate cancer: A decision analysis. *JAMA, 304*(21), 2373–2380.

3. P. Albertsen. (2008). Should patients consider active surveillance? *Cancer, 112*, 2631–2634.

4. Y. Wong, N. Mitra, G. Hudes, R. Localio, J. Schwartz, F. Wan, et al. (2006). Survival associated with treatment vs observation of localized prostate cancer in elderly men. *JAMA, 296*, 2683–2693.

5. W. Shappley III, S. Kenfield, J. Kasperzyk, W. Qiu, M. Stampfer, M. Sanda, and J. Chan. (2009). Prospective study of determinants and outcomes of deferred treatment or watchful waiting among men with prostate cancer in a nationwide cohort. *Journal of Clinical Oncology.* doi:10.1200/JCO.2008.21.2613.

6. L. Klotz. (2005). Active surveillance for good risk prostate cancer: Rationale, method, and results. *Canadian Journal of Urology, 12*(Suppl. 2), 21–24.

7. O. Bratt. (2006). Watching the face of Janus: Active surveillance as a strategy to reduce overtreatment for localized prostate cancer. *European Urology, 50,* 410–412.

8. B. Davison, J. Oliffe, T. Pickles, and L. Mroz. (2009). Factors influencing men undertaking active surveillance for the management of low-risk prostate cancer. *Oncology Nursing Forum, 36*(1), 89–96.

9. D. Bailey, M. Mishel, M. Belyea, J. Stewart, and J. Mohler. (2004). Uncertainty intervention for watchful waiting in prostate cancer. *Cancer Nursing, 27,* 339–346.

10. A. Zietman, H. Thakral, L. Wilson, and P. Schellhammer. (2001). Conservative management of prostate cancer in the prostate specific antigen era: The incidence and time course of subsequent therapy. *Journal of Urology, 166*(5), 1702–1706.

11. R. van den Bergh, M. Essink-Bot, M. Roobol, F. Schroder, C. Bangma, and E. Steyerberg. (2010). Do anxiety and distress increase during active surveillance for low risk prostate cancer? *Journal of Urology, 183,* 1786–1791.

12. R. van den Bergh, M. Essink-Bot, M. Roobol, T. Wolters, F. Schroder, C. Bangma, and E. Steyerberg. (2009). Anxiety and distress during active surveillance for early prostate cancer. *Cancer, 115,* 3868–3878.

13. K. Burnet, C. Parker, D. Dearnaley, C. Brewin, and M. Watson. (2007). Does active surveillance for men with localized prostate cancer carry psychological morbidity? *BJU International, 100,* 540–543.

14. D. Bailey, M. Wallace, and M. Mishel. (2007). Watching, waiting and uncertainty in prostate cancer. *Journal of Clinical Nursing, 16,* 734–741.

15. J. Daubenmier, G. Weidner, R. Marlin, L. Crutchfield, S. Dunn-Emke, C. Chi, P. Carrol, and D. Ornish. (2006). Lifestyle and health-related quality of life of men with prostate cancer managed with active surveillance. *Urology, 67,* 125–130.

16. J. Oliffe, B. Davison, T. Pickles, and L. Mroz. (2009). The self-management of uncertainty among men undertaking active surveillance for low-risk prostate cancer. *Qualitative Health Research, 19*(4), 432–443.

CHAPTER 5

1. J. Hu, X. Gu, S. Lipsitz, M. Barry, A. D'Amico, A. Weinberg, and N. Keating. (2009). Comparative effectiveness of minimally invasive vs open radical prostatectomy. *JAMA, 302*(14), 1557–1564.

2. R. Coelho, S. Chauhan, K. Palmer, B. Rocco, M. Patel, and V. Patel. (2009). Robotic-assisted radical prostatectomy: A review of current outcomes. *BJU International, 104,* 1428–1435.

3. K. Stitzenberg, Y. Wong, M. Nielsen, B. Egleston, and R. Uzzo. (2011). Trends in radical prostatectomy: Centralization, robotics, and access to urologic cancer care. *Cancer*. doi:10.1002/cncr.26274.

4. S. Herrell and J. Smith. (2005). Robotic-assisted laparoscopic prostatectomy: What is the learning curve? *Urology, 66*(Suppl. 5A), 105–107.

5. P. Carroll, P. Albertsen, and J. Smith. (2006). Volume of major surgeries performed by recent and more senior graduates from North American urology training programs. Paper presented at the annual meeting of the American Urological Society, Atlanta, GA.

6. V. Ficarra, G. Novara, W. Artibani, A. Cestari, A. Galfano, M. Graefen, et al. (2009). Retropubic, laparoscopic, and robot-assisted radical prostatectomy: A systematic review and cumulative analysis of comparative studies. *European Urology, 55*, 1037–1063.

7. F. Schroek, T. Krupski, L. Sun, D. Albala, M. Price, T. Polascik, et al. (2008). Satisfaction and regret after open retropubic or robot-assisted laparoscopic radical prostatectomy. *European Urology, 54*, 785–793.

8. J. Burt, K. Caelli, K. Moore, and M. Anderson. (2005). Radical prostatectomy: Men's experiences and postoperative needs. *Journal of Clinical Nursing, 14*, 883–890.

9. L. Ribeiro, C. Prota, C. Gomes, J. de Bessa Jr., M. Boldarine, M. Dall'Oglio, et al. (2010). Long-term effect of early postoperative pelvic floor biofeedback on continence in men undergoing radical prostatectomy: A prospective, randomized, controlled trial. *Journal of Urology, 184*, 1034–1039.

10. J. Lee, K. Hersey, C. Lee, and N. Fleshner. (2005). Climacturia following radical prostatectomy: Prevalence and risk factors. *Journal of Urology, 176*, 2562–2565.

11. A. Nillson, S. Carlsson, E. Johansson, M. Jonsson, C. Adding, T. Nyberg, et al. (2011). Orgasm-associated urinary incontinence and sexual life after radical prostatectomy. *Journal of Sexual Medicine*. doi:10.1111/j.1743-6109.2011.02347.x

12. H. Borchers, B. Brehmer, R. Kirschner-Hermanns, T. Reineke, L. Tietze, and G. Jakse. (2006). Erectile function after non-nerve-sparing radical prostatectomy: Fact or fiction? *Urologica Internationalis, 76*, 213–218.

13. A. Levinson, H. Lavery, N. Ward, L. Su, and C. Pavlovich. (2011). Is a return to baseline sexual function possible? An analysis of sexual function outcomes following laparoscopic radical prostatectomy. *World Journal of Urology, 29*, 29–34.

14. J. Mulhall. (2009). Defining and reporting erectile function outcomes after radical prostatectomy: Challenges and misconceptions. *Journal of Urology, 181*, 462–471.

15. J. Mulhall. (2008). *Saving your sex life: A guide for men with prostate cancer.* Munster, IN: Hilton Publishing Company, 97.

16. K. Gannon, M. Guerro-Blanco, A. Patel, and P. Abel. (2010). Re-constructing masculinity following radical prostatectomy for prostate cancer. *The Aging Male, 13*(4), 258–264.

17. G. Bronner, S. Shefi, and G. Raviv. (2010). Sexual dysfunction after radical prostatectomy: Treatment failure of treatment delay. *Journal of Sex and Marital Therapy, 36*, 421–429.

18. D. Moskovic, O. Mohamed, K. Sathyamoorthy, B. Miles, R. Link, L. Lipschultz, and M. Khera. (2010). The female factor: Predicting compliance with

a post-prostatectomy erectile preservation program. *Journal of Sexual Medicine, 7,* 3659–3665.

19. J. Mayes, V. Mouraview, M. Tsivian, T. Krupski, C. Donnatucci, and T. Polascik. (2009). Concordance in the perception of couples recovering from primary surgical treatment of prostate cancer. *International Journal of Impotence Research, 21,* 253–260.

20. T. Mason. (2005). Information needs of wives of men following prostatectomy. *Oncology Nursing Forum, 32*(3), 557–563.

CHAPTER 6

1. P. Fransson. (2010). Fatigue in prostate cancer patients treated with external beam radiotherapy: A prospective 5-year long-term patient-reported evaluation. *Journal of Cancer Research and Therapeutics, 6*(4), 516–520.

2. P. Poirier. (2011). The impact of fatigue on role functioning during radiation therapy. *Oncology Nursing Forum, 38*(4), 457–465.

3. A. Kyrdalen, A. Dahl, E. Hernes, E. Hem, and S. Fossa. (2010). Fatigue in prostate cancer survivors treated with definitive radiotherapy and LHRH analogs. *The Prostate, 70,* 1480–1489.

4. R. Segal, R. Reid, K. Courneya, R. Sigal, G. Kenny, D. Prud'Homme, et al. (2009). Randomized controlled trial of resistance or aerobic exercise in men receiving radiation therapy for prostate cancer. *Journal of Clinical Oncology, 27,* 344–351.

5. K. Mustian, L. Peppone, T. Darling, O. Palesh, C. Heckler, and G. Morrow. (2009). A 4-week home-based aerobic and resistance exercise program during radiation therapy: A pilot randomized clinical trial. *Journal of Supportive Oncology, 9,* 158–167.

6. C. Beard, W. Stason, Q. Wang, J. Manola, E. Dean-Clower, J. Dusek, et al. (2011). Effects of complementary therapies on clinical outcomes in patients being treated with radiation therapy for prostate cancer. *Cancer, 117,* 96–102.

7. A. Hanlon, D. Watkins Bruner, R. Peter, and G. Hanks. (2001). Quality of life study in prostate cancer patients treated with three-dimensional conformal radiation therapy: Comparing late bowel and bladder quality of life symptoms to that of the normal population. *International Journal of Radiation Oncology and Biological Physics, 49,* 51–59.

8. H. Geinitz, R. Thamm, C. Scholz, C. Heinrich, N. Prause, S. Kerndl, et al. (2010). Longitudinal analysis of quality of life in patients receiving conformal radiation therapy for prostate cancer. *Strahlenther Onkologie, 186,* 46–52.

9. S. Namiki, T. Satoh, S. Baba, H. Ishiyama, K. Hayakawa, S. Saito, and Y. Arai. (2006). Quality of life after brachytherapy or radical prostatectomy for localized prostate cancer: A prospective longitudinal study. *Urology, 68,* 1230–1236.

10. G. Huang, N. Sadetsky, and D. Penson. (2010). Health related quality of life for men treated for localized prostate cancer with long-term followup. *Journal of Urology, 183,* 2206–2212.

11. C. Beard. (2005). The risk of bladder, bowel, and sexual dysfunction after radiation therapy: What the data tell us and how we can use it to counsel our patients. *Cancer Journal, 11*(2), 106–109.

12. H. Geinitz, F. Zimmerman, R. Thamm, C. Erber, T. Muller, M. Keller, et al. (2006). Late rectal symptoms and quality of life after conformal radiation therapy for prostate cancer. *Radiotherapy and Oncology, 79*, 341–347.

13. M. Pinkawa, R. Holy, M. Piroth, K. Fishedick, S. Schaar, D. Szekely-Orban, and M. Eble. (2010). Consequential late effects after radiotherapy for prostate cancer: A prospective longitudinal quality of life study. *Radiation Oncology, 5*, 27.

14. M. Pinkawa, M. Piroth, K. Fishedick, S. Nussen, J. Klotz, R. Holy, and M. Eble. (2009). Self-assessed bowel toxicity after external beam radiotherapy for prostate cancer: Predictive factors on irritative symptoms, incontinence and rectal bleeding. *Radiation Oncology, 4* (36). doi:10.1186/1748-717X-4-36.

15. L. Incrocci. (2006). Sexual function after external-beam radiotherapy for prostate cancer: What do we know? *Critical Reviews in Oncology/Hematology, 57*, 165–173.

16. L. Incrocci, K. Slob, and P. Levendag. (2002). Sexual (dys)function after radiotherapy for prostate cancer: A review. *International Journal of Radiation Oncology and Biologic Physics, 52*(3), 681–693.

17. N. Stone and R. Stock. (2007). Long-term urinary, sexual, and rectal morbidity in patients treated with Iodine-125 prostate brachytherapy followed up for a minimum of 5 years. *Urology, 69*, 338–342.

18. G. van der Wielen, W. van Putten, and L. Incrocci. (2007). Sexual function after three-dimensional conformal radiotherapy for prostate cancer: Results from a dose-escalation trial. *International Journal of Radiation Oncology and Biologic Physics, 68*(2), 479–484.

19. L. Forbat, I. White, S. Marshall-Lucette, and D. Kelly. (2011). Discussing the sexual consequences of treatment in radiotherapy and urology consultations with couples affected by prostate cancer. *BJU International.* doi:10.1111/j.1464-410X.2011.10257.x.

20. L. Incrocci, W. Hop, and K. Slob. (2003). Efficacy of sildenafil in an open-label study as a continuation of a double-blind study in the treatment of erectile dysfunction after radiotherapy for prostate cancer. *Urology, 62*, 116–120.

21. J. Schiff, N. Bar-Chama, J. Cesaretti, and R. Stock. (2006). Early use of phosphodiesterase inhibitor after brachytherapy restores and preserves erectile function. *BJU International, 98*, 1255–1258.

22. J. Michalski, S. Mutic, J. Eichling, and S. Ajmed. (2003). Radiation exposure to family and household members after prostate brachytherapy. *International Journal of Radiation Oncology and Biological Physics, 56*(3), 764–768.

23. T. Mason. (2008). Wives of men with prostate brachytherapy: Perceived information needs and degree of being met. *Cancer Nursing, 31*(1), 32–37.

24. J. Grocela, T. Mauceri, and A. Zietman, A. (2005). New life after prostate brachytherapy? Considering the fertile female partner of the brachytherapy patient. *BJU International, 96*, 781–782.

CHAPTER 7

1. J. Robinson, B. Donnelly, J. Saliken, B. Weber, S. Ernst, and J. Rewcastle. (2002). Quality of life and sexuality of men with prostate cancer 3 years after cryosurgery. *Urology, 60*(Suppl. 2A), 12–18.

2. S. Asterling and D. Greene. (2008). Prospective evaluation of sexual function in patients receiving cryosurgery as a primary radical treatment for localized prostate cancer. *BJU International, 103*, 788–792.

3. G. Onik, P. Narauan, D. Vaughn, M. Dineen, and R. Brunelle. (2002). Focal "nerve sparing" cryosurgery for treatment of primary prostate cancer: A new approach to preserving potency. *Urology, 60*, 109–114.

4. D. Ellis, T. Manny Jr., and J. Rewcastle. (2007). Cryoablation as primary treatment for localized prostate cancer followed by penile rehabilitation. *Urology, 69*, 306–310.

5. S. Wilt and C. Mason. (2007). *Cryotherapy for localized prostate cancer* [Review]. The Cochrane Collection, issue 4. Accessed at www.thecochranelibrary.com.

6. R. Ganzer and A. Blana. (2010). Do we have enough evidence to recommend the routine use of high-intensity focused ultrasound for the primary and salvage treatment of prostate cancer? *European Urology, 58*, 816–818.

7. H. Lukka, T. Waldron, J. Chin, L. Mayhew, P. Warde, E. Winquist, et al. (2011). High-intensity focused ultrasound for prostate cancer: A systematic review. *Clinical Oncology, 23*, 117–127.

8. M. Warmuth, T. Johansson, and P. Mad. (2010). Systematic review of the efficacy and safety of high-intensity focused ultrasound for the primary and salvage treatment of prostate cancer. *European Urology, 58*, 803–815.

9. R. Popert. (2011). High-intensity focused ultrasound. *Clinical Oncology, 23*, 114–116.

10. J. Efstathiou, A. Torfimov, and A. Zietman. (2009). Life, liberty, and the pursuit of protons: An evidence-based review of the role of particle therapy in the treatment of prostate cancer. *Cancer Journal, 15*(4), 312–318.

11. M. Brada, M. Pijls-Johannesma, and D. De Ruysscher. (2009). Current clinical evidence for proton therapy. *Cancer Journal, 15*, 319–324.

12. J. Coen and A. Zietman. (2009). Proton radiation for localized prostate cancer. *National Review of Urology, 6*, 324–330.

13. N. Townsend, B. Huth, W. Ding, B. Garber, M. Mooreville, S. Arrigo, et al. (2011). Acute toxicity after CyberKnife-delivered hypofractionated radiotherapy for treatment of prostate cancer. *American Journal of Clinical Oncology, 34*, 6–10.

14. G. Morgia and C. De Renzis. (2009). CyberKnife in the treatment of prostate cancer: A revolutionary system. *European Urology, 56*, 40–42.

15. A. Katz. (2010). CyberKnife radiosurgery for prostate cancer. *Technology in Cancer Research and Treatment, 9*(5), 463–472.

16. C. Moore, D. Pendse, and M. Emberton. (2009). Photodynamic therapy for prostate cancer: A review of current status and future promise. *Nature Clinical Practice Urology, 6*(10), 18–30.

17. H. Ahmed, C. Moore, and M. Emberton. (2009). Minimally-invasive technologies in uro-oncology: The role of cryotherapy, HIFU and photodynamic therapy in whole gland and focal therapy of localized prostate cancer. *Surgical Oncology, 18,* 219–232.

18. N. Arumainayagam, C. Moore, H. Ahmed, and M. Emberton. (2010). Photodynamic therapy for ablation of the prostate. *World Journal of Urology, 28,* 571–576.

19. W. Demark-Wahnefried and M. Moyad. (2007). Dietary intervention in the management of prostate cancer. *Current Opinion in Urology, 17,* 168–174.

20. J. Kellog Parsons, V. Newman, J. Mohler, J. Pierce, S. Flatt, K. Messer, and J. Marshall. (2009). Dietary intervention after definitive therapy for localized prostate cancer: Results from a pilot study. *Canadian Journal of Urology, 16*(3), 4648–4654.

21. J. Carmody, B. Loendzki, G. Reed, V. Andersen, and P. Rosenzweig. (2008). A dietary intervention for recurrent prostate cancer after definitive primary treatment: Results of a randomized pilot trial. *Urology, 72,* 1324–1328.

22. L. Mroz, G. Chapman, J. Oliffe, and J. Bottorf. (2011). Men, food, and prostate cancer: Gender influences on men's diets. *American Journal of Men's Health, 5*(2), 177–187.

23. K. Kullberg, A. Aberg, A. Bjorkland, J. Ekblad, and B. Sidenvall. (2008). Daily eating events among co-living and single-living diseased older men. *Journal of Nutrition, Health and Aging, 12,* 176–182.

24. V. Helgeson, S. Novak, S. Lepore, and D. Eton. (2004). Spousal social control efforts: Relations to health behavior and well-being among men with prostate cancer. *Journal of Social and Personal Relationships, 21,* 53–68.

25. J. Satia, J. Walsh, and R. Pruthi. (2009). Health behavior change in white and African American prostate cancer survivors. *Cancer Nursing, 32*(2), 107–117.

26. A. Ponholzer, G. Struhal, and S. Madersbacher. (2003). Frequent use of complementary medicine by prostate cancer patients. *European Urology, 43,* 604–608.

27. W. Demark-Wahnefried and M. Moyad. (2007). Dietary intervention in the management of prostate cancer. *Current Opinion in Urology, 17,* 168–174.

28. World Cancer Research Fund and American Institute for Cancer Research. (2007). *Food, nutrition, physical activity and the prevention of cancer: A global perspective.* Washington, DC: Authors.

CHAPTER 8

1. A. Stephanson, M. Kattan, J. Eastham, Z. Dotan, F. Bianoc Jr., H. Lilja, and P. Scardino. (2006). Defining biochemical recurrence of prostate cancer after radical prostatectomy: A proposal for a standardized definition. *Journal of Clinical Oncology, 24,* 3973–3978.

2. K. Tzou, W. Tan, and S. Buskirk. (2011). Treatment of men with rising prostate-specific antigen levels following radical prostatectomy. *Expert Reviews in Anticancer Therapies, 11.* doi:10.1586/ERA.10.210.

3. A. Raldow, D. Hamstra, S. Kim, and J. Yu. (2011). Adjuvant radiotherapy after radical prostatectomy: Evidence and analysis. *Cancer Treatment Reviews, 37,* 89–96.

4. Tzou, Tan, and Buskirk. (2011).

5. C. Boukaram and J. Hannoun-Levi. (2010). Management of prostate cancer recurrence after definitive radiation therapy. *Cancer Treatment Reviews, 36,* 91–100.

6. J. Cox and J. Busby. (2009). Salvage therapy for prostate cancer recurrence after radiation therapy. *Current Urology Reports, 10,* 199–205.

7. M. Kimura, V. Mouraviev, M. Tsivian, J. Mayes, T. Satoh, and T. Polascik. (2009). Current salvage methods for recurrent prostate cancer after failure of primary radiotherapy. *BJU International, 105,* 191–201.

8. C. Leonardo, G. Simone, R. Papalia, G. Franco, S. Guaglianone, and M. Gallucci. (2009). Salvage radical prostatectomy for recurrent prostate cancer after radiation therapy. *International Journal of Urology, 16,* 584–586.

9. Cox and Busby. (2009).

10. Cox and Busby. (2009).

11. T. Uchida, S. Shoji, M. Nakano, S. Hongo, M. Nitta, Y. Usui, and Y. Nagata. (2010). High-intensity focused ultrasound as salvage therapy for patients with recurrent prostate cancer after external mean radiation, brachytherapy or proton therapy. *BJU International, 107,* 378–382.

12. C. Boukaram and J. Hannoun-Levi. (2010). Management of prostate cancer recurrence after definitive radiation therapy. *Cancer Treatment Reviews, 36,* 91–100.

13. J. Pendleton, W. Tan, S. Anai, M. Chang, W. Hou, K. Shivcrick, and C. Rosser. (2008). Phase II trial of isoflavone in prostate-specific antigen recurrent prostate cancer after previous local therapy. *BMC Cancer, 8,* 132; F. Schröder, M. Roobol, E. Boevé, R. de Mutsert, S. Zuijdgeest-van Leeuwen, I. Kersen, M. Wildhagen, and A. van Helvoort. (2005). Randomised, double blind, placebo-controlled crossover study in men with prostate cancer and rising PSA: effectiveness of dietary supplement. *European Urology, 48,* 922–930.

14. U. Vaishampayan, M. Hussain, M. Banerjee, S. Seren, F. Sarkcr, J. Fontana, et al. (2007). Lycopene and soy isoflavones in the treatment of prostate cancer. *Nutrition and Cancer, 59,* 1–7.

15. A. Pantuck, J. Leppert, N. Zomordian, W. Aronson, J. Hong, R. Barnard, et al. (2006). Phase II study of pomegranate juice for men with rising prostate-specific antigen following surgery or radiation for prostate cancer. *Clinical Cancer Research, 12,* 4018–4026.

16. K. Tzou, W. Tan, and S. Buskirk. (2011). Treatment of men with rising prostate-specific antigen levels following radical prostatectomy. *Expert Reviews in Anticancer Therapies, 11.* doi:10.1586/ERA.10.210.

17. S. Kenfield, M. Stampfer, J. Chan, and E. Giovannucci. (2011). Smoking and prostate cancer survival and recurrence. *JAMA, 305,* 2548–2555.

18. C. Joshu, A. Mondul, C. Meinhold, E. Humphreys, M. Han, P. Walsh, and E. Platz. (2011). Cigarette smoking and prostate cancer recurrence after prostatectomy. *Journal of the National Cancer Institute, 103,* 835–838.

19. C. Joshu, A. Mondul, A. Menke, C. Meinhold, M. Han, E. Humphreys, et al. (2011). Weight gain is associated with an increased risk of prostate cancer recurrence after prostatectomy in the PSA era. *Cancer Prevention Research, 4,* 544–551.

20. Y. Hong, J. Hu, A. Paciorek, S. Knight, and P. Carroll. (2010). Impact of radical prostatectomy positive surgical margins on fear of cancer recurrence: Results from CaPSURE. *Urologic Oncology: Seminars and Original Investigations, 28,* 268–273.

21. K. Bellizzi, D. Latini, J. Cowan, J. DuChane, and P. Carroll. (2008). Fear of recurrence, symptom burden, and health-related quality of life in men with prostate cancer. *Urology, 72,* 1269–1273.

22. S. Hart, D. Latini, J. Cowan, and P. Carroll. (2008). Fear of recurrence, treatment satisfaction, and quality of life after radical prostatectomy for prostate cancer. *Supportive Care in Cancer, 16,* 161–169.

23. S. Simard, J. Simard, and H. Ivers. (2010). Fear of cancer recurrence: Specific profiles and nature of intrusive thoughts. *Journal of Cancer Survivorship, 4,* 361–371.

CHAPTER 9

1. A. Jonsson, G. Uas, and C. Bertero. (2009). Mens' experience of their life situation when diagnosed with advanced prostate cancer. *European Journal of Oncology Nursing, 13,* 268–273.

2. C. Ryan and E. Small. (2005). Early versus delayed androgen deprivation for prostate cancer: New fuel for an old debate. *Journal of Clinical Oncology, 23,* 8225–8231.

3. W. Dale, J. Hemmerich, K. Bylow, S. Mohile, M. Mullaney, and W. Stadler. (2009). Patient anxiety about prostate cancer independently predicts early initiation of androgen deprivation therapy for biochemical recurrence in older men: A prospective cohort study. *Journal of Clinical Oncology, 27,* 1557–1563.

4. M. Bhandari, J. Crook, and M. Hussain. (2005). Should intermittent androgen deprivation be used in routine clinical practice? *Journal of Clinical Oncology, 23,* 8212–8218.

5. G. Lu-Yao, P. Albertsen, D. Moore, W. Shih, Y. Lin, R. DiPaolo, and S. Yao. (2008). Survival following primary androgen deprivation therapy among men with localized prostate cancer. *JAMA, 300,* 173–181.

6. Y. Wong, S. Freeland, B. Egleston, N. Vapiwala, R. Uzzo, and K. Armstrong. (2009). The role of primary androgen deprivation therapy in localized prostate cancer. *European Urology, 56,* 609–616.

7. J. Kawakami, M. Meng, N. Sadetsky, D. Latini, J. Duchane, P. Carroll, and CaPSURE Investigators. (2006). Changing patterns of pelvic lymphadenectomy for prostate cancer: Results from CaPSURE. *Journal of Urology, 176,* 1382–1386.

8. V. Shahinian, Y. Kuo, J. Freeman, E. Oriheuela, and J. Goodwin. (2007). Characteristics of urologists predict the use of androgen deprivation therapy for prostate cancer. *Journal of Clinical Oncology, 25,* 5359–5365.

9. C. Weight, E. Klein, and J. Jones. (2008). Androgen deprivation falls as orchiectomy rates rise after changes in reimbursement in the U.S. Medicare population. *Cancer, 112,* 2195–2201.

10. H. Harrod. (2005). An essay on desire. *Journal of the American Medical Association, 289,* 813–814.

11. K. Park, S. Lee, and B. Chung. (2011). The effects of long-term androgen deprivation therapy on penile length in patients with prostate cancer: A single-center,

prospective, open-label, observational study. *Journal of Sexual Medicine.* doi:10.1111/ j.1743-6109.2011.02364.x.

12. J. Harrington, E. Jones, and T. Badger. (2009). Body image perceptions in men with prostate cancer. *Oncology Nursing Forum, 36,* 167–172.

13. L. Navon and A. Morag. (2003). Advanced prostate cancer patients' relationships with their spouses following hormonal therapy. *European Journal of Oncology Nursing, 7,* 73–80.

14. S. Elliott, D. Latini, L. Walker, R. Wassersug, J. Robinson, and the ADT Survivorship Working Group. (2010). Androgen deprivation therapy for prostate cancer: Recommendations to improve patient and partner quality of life. *Journal of Sexual Medicine.* doi:10.1111/j.1743-6109.2010.0.1902.x.

15. R. Wassersug. (2008). Mastering emasculation. *Journal of Clinical Oncology.* doi:10.1200/JCO.2008.20.1947.

16. C. DiBlasio, J. Malcolm, I. Derweesh, J. Womack, M. Kincade, J. Mancini, et al. (2008). Patterns of sexual and erectile dysfunction and response to treatment in patients receiving androgen deprivation therapy for prostate cancer. *BJU International, 102,* 39–43.

17. C. Engstrom. (2005). Hot flash experience in men with prostate cancer: A concept analysis. *Oncology Nursing Forum, 32,* 1043–1048.

18. J. Frisk. (2010). Managing hot flushes in men after prostate cancer: A systematic review. *Maturitas, 65,* 15–22.

19. E. Winters Ulloa, R. Salup, S. Patterson, and P. Jacobsen. (2009). Relationship between hot flashes and distress in men receiving androgen deprivation therapy for prostate cancer. *Psycho-Oncology, 18,* 598–605.

20. Frisk. (2010).

21. T. Beer, M. Benavides, S. Emmons, M. Hayes, G. Liu, M. Garzotto, et al. (2010). Acupuncture for hot flashes in patients with prostate cancer. *Urology, 76,* 1182–1188.

22. G. Di Lorenzo, R. Autorino, and S. De Placido. (2005). Management of gynaecomastia in patients with prostate cancer: A systematic review. *Lancet Oncology, 6,* 972–979.

23. J. Harrington, E. Jones, and T. Badger. (2009). Body image perceptions in men with prostate cancer. *Oncology Nursing Forum, 36,* 167–172.

24. J. Harrington and T. Badger. (2009). Body image and quality of life in men with prostate cancer. *Cancer Nursing, 32,* E1–E7.

25. Navon and Morag. (2003).

26. M. Grossman and J. Zajac. (2011). Androgen deprivation therapy in men with prostate cancer: How should the side effects be monitored and treated? *Clinical Endocrinology, 74,* 289–293.

27. M. Cherrier, S. Aubin, and C. Higano. (2009). Cognitive and mood changes in men undergoing intermittent combined androgen blockade for non-metastatic prostate cancer. *Psycho-Oncology, 18,* 237–247.

28. N. Timilshina, H. Breunis, and S. Alinhai. (2011). Impact of androgen deprivation therapy on depressive symptoms in men with nonmetastatic prostate cancer. *Cancer.* doi:10.1002/cncr.26477; W. Piril, J. Greer, M. Goode, and M. Smith. (2007). Prospective study of depression and fatigue in men with advanced prostate cancer receiving hormone therapy. *Psycho-Oncology, 17,* 148–153.

29. Cherrier, Aubin, and Higano. (2009).

30. V. Shahinian, Y. Kuo, J. Freeman, and J. Goodwin. (2006). Risk of the "androgen deprivation syndrome" in men receiving androgen deprivation for prostate cancer. *Archives of Internal Medicine, 166*, 465–471.

CHAPTER 10

1. K. Cox. (2000). Enhancing cancer clinical trial management: Recommendations from a qualitative study of trial participants' experiences. *Psycho-Oncology, 9*, 314–322.

2. K. Featherstone and J. Donovan. (2002). "Why don't they just tell me straight, why allocate it?": The struggle to make sense of participating in a randomized controlled trial. *Social Science and Medicine, 55*, 709–719.

3. J. Stryker, R. Wray, K. Emmons, E. Winer, and G. Demetri. (2006). Understanding the decisions of cancer clinical trial participants to enter research studies: Factors associated with informed consent, patient satisfaction, and decisional regret. *Patient Education and Counseling, 63*, 104–109.

4. R. Wray, E. Stryker, E. Winer, G. Demetri, and K. Emmons. (2007). Do cancer patients fully understand clinical trial participation? A pilot study to assess informed consent and patient expectations. *Journal of Cancer Education, 22*, 21–24.

5. C. Grant, K. Cissna, and L. Rosenfeld. (2000). Patients' perceptions of physicians communication and outcomes of the accrual to trial process. *Health Communication, 12*(1), 23–29.

6. S. Eggly, T. Albrecht, F. Harper, T. Foster, M. Franks, and J. Ruckdeschel. (2008). Oncologists' recommendations of clinical trial participation to patients. *Patient Education and Counseling, 70*, 143–148.

7. T. Albrecht, S. Eggly, M. Gleason, F. Harper, T. Foster, A. Peterson, et al. (2008). Influence of clinical communication on patient's decision making on participation in clinical trials. *Journal of Clinical Oncology, 26*, 2666–2673.

8. Cox. (2000).

9. J. Jones, J. Nyhof-Young, J. Moric, A. Friedman, W. Wells, and P. Catton. (2006). Identifying motivations and barriers to patient participation in clinical trials. *Journal of Cancer Education, 21*, 237–242.

10. M. Buss, L. DuBenske, S. Dinauer, D. Gustafson, F. McTavish, and J. Cleary. (2008). Patient/caregiver influences for declining participation in supportive oncology trials. *Journal of Supportive Oncology, 6*, 168–174.

11. L. Yoder, T. O'Rourke, A. Etnyre, D. Spears, and T. Brown. (1997). Expectations and experiences of patients with cancer participating in Phase 1 clinical trials. *Oncology Nursing Forum, 24*(5), 891–896.

12. K. Cox and M. Avis. (1996). Psychosocial aspects of participation in early anticancer drug trials: Report of a pilot study. *Cancer Nursing, 19*(3), 177–186.

13. Available at www.johnshopkinshealthalerts.com/alerts/prostate_disorders/clinical_trials_3823-1.html.

CHAPTER 11

1. D. Feldman-Stewart, M. Brundage, and C. Tishelman. (2005). A conceptual framework for patient-professional communication: An application to the cancer context. *Psycho-Oncology, 14,* 801–809.
2. R. Ruiz-Moral, E. Perez Rodriguez, L. Perula, and J. de la Torre. (2006). Physician-patient communication: A study on the observed behaviours of specialty physicians and the ways their patients perceive them. *Patient Education and Counseling, 64,* 242–248.
3. R. Borgers, P. Mullen, R. Meertens, M. Rijken, G. Eussen, I. Plagge, et al. (1993). The information-seeking behavior of cancer outpatients: A description of the situation. *Patient Education and Counseling, 22,* 35–46.
4. S. Thorne, G. Hislop, and V. Oglov. (2009). Time-related communication skills from the cancer patient perspective. *Psycho-Oncology, 18,* 500–507.
5. U. Boehmer and J. Clark. (2001). Communication about prostate cancer between men and their wives. *Journal of Family Practice, 50*(3), 226–231.
6. L. Song, L. Northouse, L. Zhang, T. Braun, B. Cimprich, D. Ronis, and D. Mood. (2010). Study of dyadic communication in couples managing prostate cancer: A longitudinal perspective. *Psycho-Oncology.* Retrieved on line from wileyonlinelibrary.com. doi:10.1002/pon.1861.
7. S. Manne, H. Badr, T. Zaider, C. Nelson, and D. Kissane. (2010). Cancer-related communication, relationship intimacy, and psychological distress among couples coping with localized prostate cancer. *Journal of Cancer Survivorship, 4,* 74–85.
8. A. Katz. (2009). *Woman cancer sex.* Pittsburgh, PA: Hygeia Media.
9. E. Gilbert, J. Ussher, and J. Perz. (2010). Renegotiating sexuality and intimacy in the context of cancer: The experience of carers. *Archives of Sexual Behavior, 39,* 998–1009.
10. A. Beck, J. Robinson, and L. Carlson. (2009). Sexual intimacy in heterosexual couples after prostate cancer treatment: What we know and what we still need to learn. *Urologic Oncology: Seminars and Original Investigations, 27,* 137–143.

CHAPTER 12

1. S. Steginga, S. Occhipinti, J. Dunn, R. Gardiner, P. Heathcote, and J. Yaxley. (2000). The supportive care needs of men with prostate cancer. *Psycho-Oncology, 10,* 66–75.
2. J. Ussher, L. Kirsten, P. Butow, and M. Sandocal. (2005). What do cancer support groups provide which other supportive relationships do not? The experience of peer support groups for people with cancer. *Social Science and Medicine, 62,* 2565–2576.
3. J. Oliffe, J. Bottorff, M. McKenzie, T. Hislop, J. Gerbrandt, and V. Oglov. (2010). Prostate cancer support groups, health literacy and consumerism: Are community-based volunteers re-defining older men's health? *Health.* Accessed January 20, 2011, from www.hea.sagepub.com. doi:10.1177/1363459310364156.

4. J. Oliffe, J. Ogrodniczuk, J. Bottorf, T. Hislop, and M. Halpin. (2009). Connecting humor, health, and masculinities at prostate cancer support groups. *Psycho-Oncology, 18*, 916–926.

5. C. Krizek, C. Roberts, R. Ragan, J. Ferrara, and B. Lord. (1999). Gender and cancer support group participation. *Cancer Practice, 7*(2), 86–92.

6. S. Steginga, D. Smith, C. Pinnock, R. Metcalfe, R. Gardiner, and J. Dunn. (2006). Clinicians' attitudes to prostate cancer peer-support groups. *BJU International, 99*, 68–71.

7. J. Bottorf, J. Oliffe, M. Halpin, M. Phillips, G. McLean, and L. Mroz. (2008). Women and prostate cancer support groups: The gender connect? *Social Science and Medicine, 66*, 1217–1227.

8. G. Eysenbach, J. Powell, M. Englesakis, C. Rizo, and A. Stern. (2004). Health related virtual communities and electronic support groups: Systematic review of the effects of online peer to peer interactions. *British Medical Journal, 328*.

9. E. Im, W. Chee, Y. Liu, H. Lim, E. Guevara, H. Tsai, et al. (2007). Characteristics of cancer patients in Internet cancer support groups. *Computers, Informatics, Nursing, 25*(6), 334–343.

10. C. Seale, S. Ziebland, and J. Charteris-Blach. (2006). Gender, cancer experience and Internet use: A comparative keyword analysis of interviews and online cancer support groups. *Social Science and Medicine, 62*, 2577–2590.

11. J. Huber, A. Ihring, T. Peters, C. Huber, A. Kessler, B. Hadaschik, et al. (2010). Decision-making in localized prostate cancer: Lessons learned from an online support group. *BJU International*. doi:10.111/j.1464-410X.2010.09859.x.

12. C. Seale. (2006). Gender accommodation in online cancer support groups. *Health, 10*(3), 345–360.

13. P. Klemm and E. Wheeler. (2005). Cancer care givers online: Hope, emotional roller coaster, and physical/emotional/psychological responses. *Computers, Informatics, Nursing, 23*(1), 38–45.

14. A. Meier, E. Lyons, G. Frydman, M. Forlenza, and B. Rimer. (2007). How cancer survivors provide support on cancer-related internet mailing lists. *Journal of Medical Internet Research, 9*(2), e12.

CHAPTER 13

1. M. Shelley, C. Harrison, B. Coles, J. Stafforth, T. Wilt, and M. Mason. (2008). Chemotherapy for hormone-refractory prostate cancer [Review]. *Cochrane Database of Systematic Reviews, 4*(Art. No. CD005247). doi:10.1002/14651858.CD005247.pub2.

2. D. Vasani, D. Josephson, C. Carmichael, O. Sartor, and S. Pal. (2011). Recent advances in the therapy of castration-resistant prostate cancer: The price of progress. *Maturitas, 70*, 194–196.

3. S. Bracarda, C. Logothetis, C. Sternberg, and S. Oudard. (2011). Current and emerging treatment modalities for metastatic castration-resistant prostate cancer. *BJU International, 107*(Suppl. 2), 13–20.

4. S. Pal and O. Sartor. (2011). Current paradigms and evolving concepts in metastatic castration-resistant prostate cancer. *Asian Journal of Andrology, 13,* 683–689.

5. G. Colloca, A. Venturino, and F. Checcaglini. (2010). Patient-reported outcomes after cytotoxic chemotherapy in metastatic castration-resistant prostate cancer: A systematic review. *Cancer Treatment Reviews, 36,* 501–506.

6. J. Thompson, J. Wood, and D. Feuer. (2007). Prostate cancer: Palliative care and pain relief. *British Medical Bulletin, 83,* 341–354.

7. J. Wu, F. Meyers, and C. Evans. (2011). Palliative care in urology. *Surgical Clinics of North America, 91,* 429–444.

8. Wu, Meyers, and Evans. (2011).

9. J. Bergman, C. Saigal, K. Lorenz, J. Hanley, D. Miller, J. Gore, and M. Litwin. (2011). Hospice use and high-intensity care in men dying of prostate cancer. *Archives of Internal Medicine, 171*(3), 204–210.

CHAPTER 14

1. A. Thornton and M. Perez. (2006). Posttraumatic growth in prostate cancer survivors and their partners. *Psycho-Oncology, 15,* 285–296.

Bibliography

Albertsen, P. (2010). Further support for active surveillance in the management of low-volume, low-grade prostate cancer. *European Urology, 58*(6), 836–837. doi:10.1016/j.eururo.2010.09.003

Albertsen, P. C. (2010). Treatment of localized prostate cancer: When is active surveillance appropriate? *Nature Reviews Clinical Oncology, 7*(7), 394–400. doi:10.1038/nrclinonc.2010.63

Albertsen, P. C. (2011). When is active surveillance the appropriate treatment for prostate cancer? *Acta Oncologica* (Stockholm, Sweden), *50*(Suppl. 1), 120–126. doi:10.31 09/0284186X.2010.526634

Alongi, F., Cozzarini, C., Di Muzio, N., & Scorsetti, M. (2011). Postoperative radiotherapy in prostate cancer: Acquired certainties and still open issues; a review of recent literature. *Tumori, 97*(1), 1–8.

Antonarakis, E. S., & Armstrong, A. J. (2011). Emerging therapeutic approaches in the management of metastatic castration-resistant prostate cancer. *Prostate Cancer and Prostatic Diseases, 14*(3), 206–218. doi:10.1038/pcan.2011.24; 10.1038/pcan.2011.24

Bannuru, R. R., Dvorak, T., Obadan, N., Yu, W. W., Patel, K., Chung, M., & Ip, S. (2011). Comparative evaluation of radiation treatments for clinically localized prostate cancer: An updated systematic review. *Annals of Internal Medicine, 155*(3), 171–178. doi:10.1059/0003-4819-155-3-201108020-00347

Barry, M. (2011). Documenting the genie's escape: Robotic surgery. *Medical Care, 49*(4), 340–342. doi:10.1097/MLR.0b013e3182125d88

Beltran, H., Beer, T. M., Carducci, M. A., de Bono, J., Gleave, M., Hussain, et al. (2011). New therapies for castration-resistant prostate cancer: Efficacy and safety. *European Urology, 60*(2), 279–290. doi:10.1016/j.eururo.2011.04.038

Borin, J. F. (2011). Imaging for staging prostate cancer: Too much or not enough? *Journal of Urology, 186*(3), 779–780. doi:10.1016/j.juro.2011.07.039

Bowes, D., & Crook, J. (2011). A critical analysis of the long-term impact of brachytherapy for prostate cancer: A review of the recent literature. *Current Opinion in Urology, 21*(3), 219–224. doi:10.1097/MOU.0b013e3283449d52

Bratt, O., & Schumacher, M. C. (2011). Natural history of prostate cancer, chemo-prevention and active surveillance. *Acta Oncologica* (Stockholm, Sweden), *50*(Suppl. 1), 116–119. doi:10.3109/0284186X.2010.527369

Buchan, N. C., & Goldenberg, S. L. (2010). Intermittent androgen suppression for prostate cancer. *Nature Reviews Urology, 7*(10), 552–560. doi:10.1038/nrurol.2010.141

Capitanio, U. (2011). Contemporary management of patients with T1a and T1b prostate cancer. *Current Opinion in Urology, 21*(3), 252–256. doi:10.1097/MOU.0b013e328344e4ad

Carter, H. B. (2011). Management of low (favourable)-risk prostate cancer. *BJU International, 108*(11), 1684–1695. doi:10.1111/j.1464-410X.2010.10489.x; 10.1111/j.1464-410X.2010.10489.x

Chaussy, C. G., & Thuroff, S. F. (2011). Robotic high-intensity focused ultrasound for prostate cancer: What have we learned in 15 years of clinical use? *Current Urology Reports, 12*(3), 180–187. doi:10.1007/s11934-011-0184-2

Cheraghi-Sohi, S., & Bower, P. (2008). Can the feedback of patient assessments, brief training, or their combination, improve the interpersonal skills of primary care physicians? A systematic review. *BMC Health Services Research, 8*, 179. doi:10.1186/1472-6963-8-179

Choi, S. (2011). The role of magnetic resonance imaging in the detection of prostate cancer. *Journal of Urology, 186*(4), 1181–1182. doi:10.1016/j.juro.2011.07.046

Cooperberg, M. R., Carroll, P. R., & Klotz, L. (2011). Active surveillance for prostate cancer: Progress and promise. *Journal of Clinical Oncology: Official Journal of the American Society of Clinical Oncology, 29*(27), 3669–3676. doi:10.1200/JCO.2011.34.9738

Corona, G., Baldi, E., & Maggi, M. (2011). Androgen regulation of prostate cancer: Where are we now? *Journal of Endocrinological Investigation, 34*(3), 232–243. doi:10.3275/7501

Crook, J. (2011). The role of brachytherapy in the definitive management of prostate cancer. *Cancer Radiotherapie: Journal De La Societe Francaise De Radiotherapie Oncologique, 15*(3), 230–237. doi:10.1016/j.canrad.2011.01.004

Croswell, J. M., Kramer, B. S., & Crawford, E. D. (2011). Screening for prostate cancer with PSA testing: Current status and future directions. *Oncology* (Williston Park, NY), *25*(6), 452–460, 463.

da Silva, F. C. (2011). Intermittent hormonal therapy for prostate cancer. *Current Opinion in Urology, 21*(3), 248–251. doi:10.1097/MOU.0b013e328344f3e3

Dahm, P., Kang, D., Stoffs, T. L., & Canfield, S. E. (2011). Recovery of erectile function after robotic prostatectomy: Evidence-based outcomes. *The Urologic Clinics of North America, 38*(2), 95–103. doi:10.1016/j.ucl.2011.02.001

D'Amico, A. V. (2011). Risk-based management of prostate cancer. *New England Journal of Medicine, 365*(2), 169–171. doi:10.1056/NEJMe1103829

Davis, J. W., & Shih, Y. C. (2011). Trends in the care of radical prostatectomy in the United States from 2003 to 2006. *BJU International, 108*(1), 49–55. doi:10.1111/j.1464-410X.2011.10438.x

Dayyani, F., Gallick, G. E., Logothetis, C. J., & Corn, P. G. (2011). Novel therapies for metastatic castrate-resistant prostate cancer. *Journal of the National Cancer Institute, 103*(22), 1665–1675. doi:10.1093/jnci/djr362

Djavan, B. (2011). Editorial: Immunotherapy for prostate cancer. *Canadian Journal of Urology, 18*(4), 5763.

Duffey, B., Varda, B., & Konety, B. (2011). Quality of evidence to compare outcomes of open and robot-assisted laparoscopic prostatectomy. *Current Urology Reports, 12*(3), 229–236. doi:10.1007/s11934-011-0180-6

Elliott, S., Latini, D. M., Walker, L. M., Wassersug, R., Robinson, J. W., & ADT Survivorship Working Group. (2010). Androgen deprivation therapy for prostate cancer: Recommendations to improve patient and partner quality of life. *Journal of Sexual Medicine, 7*(9), 2996–3010. doi:10.1111/j.1743-6109.2010.01902.x

Evans, A. J., Ryan, P., & Van derKwast, T. (2011). Treatment effects in the prostate including those associated with traditional and emerging therapies. *Advances in Anatomic Pathology, 18*(4), 281–293. doi:10.1097/PAP.0b013e318220f5b1

Faris, J. E., & Smith, M. R. (2010). Metabolic sequelae associated with androgen deprivation therapy for prostate cancer. *Current Opinion in Endocrinology, Diabetes, and Obesity, 17*(3), 240–246. doi:10.1097/MED.0b013e3283391fd1

Farooqi, A. A., & Bhatti, S. (2011). Getting personal with prostate cancer: Adding new pieces to an incomplete jigsaw puzzle. *Urologia Internationalis, 87*(2), 127–133. doi:10.1159/000327723

Filella, X., Alcover, J., & Molina, R. (2011). Active surveillance in prostate cancer: The need to standardize. *Tumour Biology: Journal of the International Society for Oncodevelopmental Biology and Medicine, 32*(5), 839–843. doi:10.1007/s13277-011-0193-2

Finley, D. S., & Belldegrun, A. S. (2011). Salvage cryotherapy for radiation-recurrent prostate cancer: Outcomes and complications. *Current Urology Reports, 12*(3), 209–215. doi:10.1007/s11934-011-0182-4

Freedland, S. J. (2011). Screening, risk assessment, and the approach to therapy in patients with prostate cancer. *Cancer, 117*(6), 1123–1135. doi:10.1002/cncr.25477

Freedman, R. A., & Garber, J. E. (2011). Family cancer history: Healthy skepticism required. *Journal of the National Cancer Institute, 103*(10), 776–777. doi:10.1093/jnci/djr142

Galvão, D. A., Taaffe, D. R., Spry, N., & Newton, R. U. (2011). Physical activity and genitourinary cancer survivorship. *Recent Results in Cancer Research. Fortschritte Der Krebsforschung. Progres Dans Les Recherches Sur Le Cancer, 186*, 217–236. doi:10.1007/978-3-642-04231-7_9

Gao, W., Bennett, M. I., Stark, D., Murray, S., & Higginson, I. J. (2010). Psychological distress in cancer from survivorship to end of life care: Prevalence, associated factors and clinical implications. *European Journal of Cancer* (Oxford, England: 1990), *46*(11), 2036–2044. doi:10.1016/j.ejca.2010.03.033

Ginzburg, S., & Albertsen, P. C. (2011). The timing and extent of androgen deprivation therapy for prostate cancer: Weighing the clinical evidence. *Endocrinology and Metabolism Clinics of North America, 40*(3), 615–623, ix. doi:10.1016/j.ecl.2011.05.005

Grace, S. L., Evindar, A., Abramson, B. L., & Stewart, D. E. (2004). Physician management preferences for cardiac patients: Factors affecting referral to cardiac rehabilitation. *Canadian Journal of Cardiology, 20*(11), 1101–1107.

Grossmann, M., & Zajac, J. D. (2011). Management of side effects of androgen deprivation therapy. *Endocrinology and Metabolism Clinics of North America, 40*(3), 655–671, x. doi:10.1016/j.ecl.2011.05.004

Gulley, J. L., & Drake, C. G. (2011). Immunotherapy for prostate cancer: Recent advances, lessons learned, and areas for further research. *Clinical Cancer Research: An Official Journal of the American Association for Cancer Research, 17*(12), 3884–3891. doi:10.1158/1078-0432.CCR-10-2656

Hammerstrom, A. E., Cauley, D. H., Atkinson, B. J., & Sharma, P. (2011). Cancer immunotherapy: Sipuleucel-T and beyond. *Pharmacotherapy, 31*(8), 813–828. doi:10.1592/phco.31.8.813

Haywood, K., Marshall, S., & Fitzpatrick, R. (2006). Patient participation in the consultation process: A structured review of intervention strategies. *Patient Education and Counseling, 63*(1–2), 12–23. doi:10.1016/j.pec.2005.10.005

Hoffman, R. M. (2011). Clinical practice: Screening for prostate cancer. *New England Journal of Medicine, 365*(21), 2013–2019. doi:10.1056/NEJMcp1103642

Hugosson, J., Stranne, J., & Carlsson, S. V. (2011). Radical retropubic prostatectomy: A review of outcomes and side-effects. *Acta Oncologica* (Stockholm, Sweden), *50*(Suppl. 1), 92–97. doi:10.3109/0284186X.2010.535848

Iczkowski, K. A., & Lucia, M. S. (2011). Current perspectives on Gleason grading of prostate cancer. *Current Urology Reports, 12*(3), 216–222. doi:10.1007/s11934-011-0181-5

Ilic, D., O'Connor, D., Green, S., & Wilt, T. J. (2011). Screening for prostate cancer: An updated Cochrane systematic review. *BJU International, 107*(6), 882–891. doi:10.1111/j.1464-410X.2010.10032.x

Kao, J., Cesaretti, J. A., Stone, N. N., & Stock, R. G. (2011). Update on prostate brachytherapy: Long-term outcomes and treatment-related morbidity. *Current Urology Reports, 12*(3), 237–242. doi:10.1007/s11934-011-0183-3

Kazzazi, A., Momtahen, S., Bruhn, A., Hemani, M., Ramaswamy, K., & Djavan, B. (2011). New findings in localized and advanced prostate cancer: AUA 2011 review. *Canadian Journal of Urology, 18*(3), 5683–5688.

Kim, H. S., & Freedland, S. J. (2010). Androgen deprivation therapy in prostate cancer: Anticipated side-effects and their management. *Current Opinion in Supportive and Palliative Care, 4*(3), 147–152. doi:10.1097/SPC.0b013e32833bd913

Klotz, L. (2011). Active surveillance for favorable risk prostate cancer: Rationale, results, and vis-à-vis focal therapy role. *Minerva Urologica e Nefrologica = the Italian Journal of Urology and Nephrology, 63*(2), 145–153.

Krakowsky, Y., Loblaw, A., & Klotz, L. (2010). Prostate cancer death of men treated with initial active surveillance: Clinical and biochemical characteristics. *Journal of Urology, 184*(1), 131–135. doi:10.1016/j.juro.2010.03.041

Lattouf, J. B., & Saad, F. (2010). Bone complications of androgen deprivation therapy: Screening, prevention, and treatment. *Current Opinion in Urology, 20*(3), 247–252. doi:10.1097/MOU.0b013e32833835be

Lee, C. H., Akin-Olugbade, O., & Kirschenbaum, A. (2011). Overview of prostate anatomy, histology, and pathology. *Endocrinology and Metabolism Clinics of North America, 40*(3), 565–575, viii–ix. doi:10.1016/j.ecl.2011.05.012

Légaré, F., Ratté, S., Stacey, D., Kryworuchko, J., Gravel, K., Graham, I. D., & Turcotte, S. (2010). Interventions for improving the adoption of shared decision making by healthcare professionals. *Cochrane Database of Systematic Reviews (Online), 5*(5), CD006732. doi:10.1002/14651858.CD006732.pub2

Lewin, S. A., Skea, Z. C., Entwistle, V., Zwarenstein, M., & Dick, J. (2001). Interventions for providers to promote a patient-centred approach in clinical consultations. *Cochrane Database of Systematic Reviews (Online), 4*(4), CD003267. doi:10.1002/14651858.CD003267

Lindner, U., Lawrentschuk, N., Schatloff, O., Trachtenberg, J., & Lindner, A. (2011). Evolution from active surveillance to focal therapy in the management of prostate cancer. *Future Oncology* (London, England), *7*(6), 775–787. doi:10.2217/fon.11.51

Loblaw, A., Zhang, L., Lam, A., Nam, R., Mamedov, A., Vesprini, D., & Klotz, L. (2010). Comparing prostate specific antigen triggers for intervention in men with stable prostate cancer on active surveillance. *Journal of Urology, 184*(5), 1942–1946. doi:10.1016/j.juro.2010.06.101

Logothetis, C. J. (2011). When "dueling technologies" are mistaken for progress. *BJU International, 107*(11), 1699–1700. doi:10.1111/j.1464-410X.2011.10243.x

Marberger, M. (2011). Is robot-assisted radical prostatectomy safer than other radical prostatectomy techniques? *European Urology, 59*(5), 699–700; discussion 701. doi:10.1016/j.eururo.2011.02.030

Mauksch, L. B., Dugdale, D. C., Dodson, S., & Epstein, R. (2008). Relationship, communication, and efficiency in the medical encounter: Creating a clinical model from a literature review. *Archives of Internal Medicine, 168*(13), 1387–1395. doi:10.1001/archinte.168.13.1387

Mazzucchelli, R., Nesseris, I., Cheng, L., Lopez-Beltran, A., Montironi, R., & Scarpelli, M. (2010). Active surveillance for low-risk prostate cancer. *Anticancer Research, 30*(9), 3683–3692.

McKenzie, P., Delahunt, B., deVoss, K., Ross, B., Tran, H., & Sikaris, K. (2011). Prostate specific antigen testing for the diagnosis of prostate cancer. *Pathology, 43*(5), 403. doi:10.1097/PAT.0b013e32834915fc

Moskovic, D. J., Miles, B. J., Lipshultz, L. I., & Khera, M. (2011). Emerging concepts in erectile preservation following radical prostatectomy: A guide for clinicians. *International Journal of Impotence Research, 23*(5), 181–192. doi:10.1038/ijir.2011.26; 10.1038/ijir.2011.26

Mostaghel, E. A., & Plymate, S. (2011). New hormonal therapies for castration-resistant prostate cancer. *Endocrinology and Metabolism Clinics of North America, 40*(3), 625–642, x. doi:10.1016/j.ecl.2011.05.013

Mottrie, A., De Naeyer, G., Novara, G., & Ficarra, V. (2011). Robotic radical prostatectomy: A critical analysis of the impact on cancer control. *Current Opinion in Urology, 21*(3), 179–184. doi:10.1097/MOU.0b013e328344e53e

Mottrie, A., Gallina, A., De Wil, P., Thuer, D., Novara, G., & Ficarra, V. (2011). Balancing continence function and oncological outcomes during robot-assisted radical prostatectomy (RARP). *BJU International, 108*(6 Pt. 2), 999–1006. doi:10.1111/j.1464-410X.2011.10529.x; 10.1111/j.1464-410X.2011.10529.x

Mulhall, J. (2009). Defining and reporting erectile function outcomes after radical prostatectomy: Challenges and misconceptions. *Journal of Urology, 181*, 462–471.

Mulhall, J. (2008). *Saving your sex life: A guide for men with prostate cancer.* Munster, IN: Hilton Publishing Company.

Nguyen, C. T., & Jones, J. S. (2011). Focal therapy in the management of localized prostate cancer. *BJU International, 107*(9), 1362–1368. doi:10.1111/j.1464-410X.2010.09975.x

Nguyen, P. L., Je, Y., Schutz, F. A., Hoffman, K. E., Hu, J. C., Parekh, A., et al. (2011). Association of androgen deprivation therapy with cardiovascular death in patients with prostate cancer: A meta-analysis of randomized trials. *JAMA: Journal of the American Medical Association, 306*(21), 2359–2366. doi:10.1001/jama.2011.1745

Oliffe, J. L., Halpin, M., Bottorff, J. L., Hislop, T. G., McKenzie, M., & Mroz, L. (2008). How prostate cancer support groups do and do not survive: British Columbian perspectives. *American Journal of Men's Health, 2*(2), 143–155. doi:10.1177/1557988307304147

Permuth-Wey, J., & Borenstein, A. R. (2009). Financial remuneration for clinical and behavioral research participation: Ethical and practical considerations. *Annals of Epidemiology, 19*(4), 280–285. doi:10.1016/j.annepidem.2009.01.004

Pickles, T., Ruether, J. D., Weir, L., Carlson, L., Jakulj, F., & SCRN Communication Team. (2007). Psychosocial barriers to active surveillance for the management of early prostate cancer and a strategy for increased acceptance. *BJU International, 100*(3), 544–551. doi:10.1111/j.1464-410X.2007.06981.x

Pierce, R., Chadiha, L. A., Vargas, A., & Mosley, M. (2003). Prostate cancer and psychosocial concerns in African American men: Literature synthesis and recommendations. *Health & Social Work, 28*(4), 302–311.

Ploussard, G., Epstein, J. I., Montironi, R., Carroll, P. R., Wirth, M., Grimm, M. O., et al. (2011). The contemporary concept of significant versus insignificant prostate cancer. *European Urology, 60*(2), 291–303. doi:10.1016/j.eururo.2011.05.006

Porche, D. (2011). Prostate cancer: Overview of screening, diagnosis and treatment. *Advance for NPs & PAs, 2*(6), 18–21; quiz 22.

Rao, J. K., Anderson, L. A., Inui, T. S., & Frankel, R. M. (2007). Communication interventions make a difference in conversations between physicians and patients: A systematic review of the evidence. *Medical Care, 45*(4), 340–349. doi:10.1097/01.mlr.0000254516.04961.d5

Reinders, M. E., Ryan, B. L., Blankenstein, A. H., van der Horst, H. E., Stewart, M. A., & van Marwijk, H. W. (2011). The effect of patient feedback on physicians' consultation skills: A systematic review. *Academic Medicine: Journal of the Association of American Medical Colleges, 86*(11), 1426–1436. doi:10.1097/ACM.0b013e3182312162

Roehrborn, C. G., & Black, L. K. (2011). The economic burden of prostate cancer. *BJU International, 108*(6), 806–813. doi:10.1111/j.1464-410X.2011.10365.x

Schmid, H. P., Fischer, C., Engeler, D. S., Bendhack, M. L., & Schmitz-Drager, B. J. (2011). Nutritional aspects of primary prostate cancer prevention. *Recent Results in Cancer Research. Fortschritte Der Krebsforschung. Progres Dans Les Recherches Sur Le Cancer, 188*, 101–107. doi:10.1007/978-3-642-10858-7_8

Schröder, F. H. (2011). Screening for prostate cancer. *European Journal of Cancer* (Oxford, England, 1990), *47*(Suppl. 3), S164–170. doi:10.1016/S0959-8049(11)70160-5

Simmons, M. N., Berglund, R. K., & Jones, J. S. (2011). A practical guide to prostate cancer diagnosis and management. *Cleveland Clinic Journal of Medicine, 78*(5), 321–331. doi:10.3949/ccjm.78a.10104

Smith, M. R. (2011). Effective treatment for early-stage prostate cancer: Possible, necessary, or both? *New England Journal of Medicine, 364*(18), 1770–1772. doi:10.1056/NEJMe1100787

Stacey, D., Bennett, C. L., Barry, M. J., Col, N. F., Eden, K. B., Holmes-Rovner, M., et al. (2011). Decision aids for people facing health treatment or screening decisions. *Cochrane Database of Systematic Reviews (Online), 10*(10), CD001431. doi:10.1002/14651858.CD001431.pub3

Stamatiou, K. N. (2011). Elderly and prostate cancer screening. *Urology Journal, 8*(2), 83–87.

Tabatabaei, S., Saylor, P. J., Coen, J., & Dahl, D. M. (2011). Prostate cancer imaging: What surgeons, radiation oncologists, and medical oncologists want to know. *AJR: American Journal of Roentgenology, 196*(6), 1263–1266. doi:10.2214/AJR.10.6263

Ramsey, S. D., Zeliadt, S. B., Fedorenko, C. R., Blough, D. K., Moinpour, C. M., Hall, I. J., et al. (2011). Patient preferences and urologist recommendations among local-stage prostate cancer patients who present for initial consultation and second opinions. *World Journal of Urology, 29*(1), 3–9. doi:10.1007/s00345-010-0602-y

Sammons, H. (2009). Ethical issues of clinical trials in children: A European perspective. *Archives of Disease in Childhood, 94*(6), 474–477. doi:10.1136/adc.2008.149898

Shaha, M., Cox, C. L., Talman, K., & Kelly, D. (2008). Uncertainty in breast, prostate, and colorectal cancer: Implications for supportive care. *Journal of Nursing Scholarship: An Official Publication of Sigma Theta Tau International Honor Society of Nursing/Sigma Theta Tau, 40*(1), 60–67. doi:10.1111/j.1547-5069.2007.00207.x

Sharifi, N., Gulley, J. L., & Dahut, W. L. (2010). An update on androgen deprivation therapy for prostate cancer. *Endocrine-Related Cancer, 17*(4), R305-315. doi:10.1677/ERC-10-0187

Sinfield, P., Baker, R., Camosso-Stefinovic, J., Colman, A. M., Tarrant, C., Mellon, J. K., et al. (2009). Men's and carers' experiences of care for prostate cancer: A narrative literature review. *Health Expectations: An International Journal of Public Participation in Health Care and Health Policy, 12*(3), 301–312. doi:10.1111/j.1369-7625.2009.00546.x

Smith, M. R. (2011). Effective treatment for early-stage prostate cancer: Possible, necessary, or both? *New England Journal of Medicine, 364*(18), 1770–1772. doi:10.1056/NEJMe1100787

Sonpavde, G., & Sternberg, C. N. (2011). Contemporary management of metastatic castration-resistant prostate cancer. *Current Opinion in Urology, 21*(3), 241–247. doi:10.1097/MOU.0b013e3283449e19

Srivastava, A., Grover, S., Sooriakumaran, P., Joneja, J., & Tewari, A. K. (2011). Robotic-assisted laparoscopic prostatectomy: A critical analysis of its impact on urinary continence. *Current Opinion in Urology, 21*(3), 185–194. doi:10.1097/MOU.0b013e3283455a21

Stacey, D., Bennett, C. L., Barry, M. J., Col, N. F., Eden, K. B., Holmes-Rovner, M., et al. (2011). Decision aids for people facing health treatment or screening decisions. *Cochrane Database of Systematic Reviews (Online), 10*(10), CD001431. doi:10.1002/14651858.CD001431.pub3

Sternberg, C. N. (2011). Novel treatments for castration-resistant prostate cancer. *European Journal of Cancer* (Oxford, England, 1990), *47*(Suppl. 3), S195-199. doi:10.1016/S0959-8049(11)70165-4

Stone, N. N. (2011). Survival after prostate brachytherapy in patients aged 60 years and younger. *BJU International, 107*(12), 1911-410X.2011.10409.x. doi:10.1111/j.1464-410X.2011.10409.x

Sturge, J., Caley, M. P., & Waxman, J. (2011). Bone metastasis in prostate cancer: Emerging therapeutic strategies. *Nature Reviews Clinical Oncology, 8*(6), 357–368. doi:10.1038/nrclinonc.2011.67

Tanaka, T., & Nakatani, T. (2011). New therapeutic strategies for castration-resistant prostate cancer. *Recent Patents on Anti-Cancer Drug Discovery, 6*(3), 373–383. doi:10.2174/157489211796957793

Thaxton, L., Emshoff, J. G., & Guessous, O. (2005). Prostate cancer support groups: A literature review. *Journal of Psychosocial Oncology, 23*(1), 25–40. doi:10.1300/J077v23n01_02

Thompson, I. M., & Klotz, L. (2010). Active surveillance for prostate cancer. *JAMA: Journal of the American Medical Association, 304*(21), 2411–2412. doi:10.1001/jama.2010.1761

Ukimura, O., Hung, A. J., & Gill, I. S. (2011). Innovations in prostate biopsy strategies for active surveillance and focal therapy. *Current Opinion in Urology, 21*(2), 115–120. doi:10.1097/MOU.0b013e3283435118

Ullen, A., Shah, C. H., & Kirkali, Z. (2011). Management of advanced prostate cancer: New drugs. *Acta Oncologica* (Stockholm, Sweden), *50*(Suppl. 1), 137–140. doi:10.3109/0284186X.2010.529458

van den Bergh, R. C., van Vugt, H. A., Korfage, I. J., Steyerberg, E. W., Roobol, M. J., Schroder, F. H., & Essink-Bot, M. L. (2010). Disease insight and treatment perception of men on active surveillance for early prostate cancer. *BJU International, 105*(3), 322–328. doi:10.1111/j.1464-410X.2009.08764.x

Venderbos, L. D., & Roobol, M. J. (2011). PSA-based prostate cancer screening: The role of active surveillance and informed and shared decision making. *Asian Journal of Andrology, 13*(2), 219–224. doi:10.1038/aja.2010.180

Walker, L. M., & Robinson, J. W. (2010). The unique needs of couples experiencing androgen deprivation therapy for prostate cancer. *Journal of Sex & Marital Therapy, 36*(2), 154–165. doi:10.1080/00926230903554552

Weber, B. A., & Sherwill-Navarro, P. (2005). Psychosocial consequences of prostate cancer: 30 years of research. *Geriatric Nursing* (New York), *26*(3), 166–175. doi:10.1016/j.gerinurse.2005.05.001

Whitson, J. M., & Carroll, P. R. (2010). Active surveillance for early-stage prostate cancer: Defining the triggers for intervention. *Journal of Clinical Oncology: Official Journal of the American Society of Clinical Oncology, 28*(17), 2807–2809. doi:10.1200/JCO.2010.28.5817

Wilson, T., & Torrey, R. (2011). Open versus robotic-assisted radical prostatectomy: Which is better? *Current Opinion in Urology, 21*(3), 200–205. doi:10.1097/MOU.0b013e32834493b3

Yang, W., & Levine, A. C. (2011). Androgens and prostate cancer bone metastases: Effects on both the seed and the soil. *Endocrinology and Metabolism Clinics of North America, 40*(3), 643–653, x. doi:10.1016/j.ecl.2011.05.001

Yates, D. R., Roupret, M., Bitker, M. O., & Vaessen, C. (2011). To infinity and beyond: The robotic toy story. *European Urology, 60*(2), 263–265. doi:10.1016/j.eururo.2011.02.039

Zandbelt, L. C., Smets, E. M., Oort, F. J., Godfried, M. H., & de Haes, H. C. (2007). Patient participation in the medical specialist encounter: Does physicians' patient-centred communication matter? *Patient Education and Counseling, 65*(3), 396–406. doi:10.1016/j.pec.2006.09.011

Index

About the Author

Anne Katz is a clinical nurse specialist at CancerCare Manitoba. She is the author of the award-winning books *Breaking the Silence on Cancer and Sexuality: A Handbook for Health Care Providers*, *Woman Cancer Sex*, and *Man Cancer Sex*. She is also the author of *Surviving after Cancer: Living the New Normal*, *Sex When You're Sick: Reclaiming Sexual Health after Illness or Injury*, and *Girl in the Know: Your Inside-and-Out Guide to Growing Up*. Dr. Katz is also the editor of *Oncology Nursing Forum*, the premier research journal published by the Oncology Nursing Society.